Sex Tips

From Men Who Ride the Sexual Frontier

Jo-Anne Baker

To my parents, who have been a constant source of love and support in my life

First published in Great Britain by Fusion Press, a division of Satin Publications Ltd.

Fusion Press
101 Southwark Street
London SE1 0JH
UK
e-mail: info@visionpaperbacks.co.uk
website: www.visionpaperbacks.com

Publisher: Sheena Dewan
Cover design © 2001 Nickolai Globe
Typeset by FiSH Books, London
Printed and bound in the UK by Biddles Ltd.

ISBN: 1-901250-85-7

Contents

Acknowledgements *vii*

1 Leaders of the Pack 1
Joseph Kramer/Mantak Chia/Stan Dale

2 Sexual Spirit 23
Willem de Ridder/Keith Hennessy/Panos Couros

3 You Sexy Thing 47
Shai Shahar/Dan Savage/Justin Case

4 Sexy is the World 67
Richard Pacheco/Jack Heidenry/Robbie Swan

5 All Kinds of People 89
Layne Winklebleck/Robert McGinley

6 That's the Way Sex Is 101
David Steinberg/Kenneth Ray Stubbs/Kerry Riley

7 Sexual Healing 119
Jules Black/David Brown/Michael Castleman/Bill O'Hanlon

8 Unchained Melody 157
Dominic Davies/George Taleporos/Eugene Moore

9 Celestial Spirit 179
Reverend Bill Huff Johnston/Rabbi Shmuley Boteach/Winton Higgins

10 The Rhythm of Life Has A Powerful Beat 195

Further Information *241*

Bibliography *245*

About the Author *247*

Acknowledgements

I would like to thank all the men in this book who have inspired me and given me their words of wisdom and depth of knowledge.

To Kimberly O'Sullivan, for her invaluable help – I would not have been able to compile this book without you.

To Esmé Holmes for her love and support.

To Annie Sprinkle and Joani Blank for their help with the project.

To the men in my life: Dhiren, Ron Tanner and Frank Morgan.

'See thou character. Give thy thoughts no tongue,
Nor any unproportioned thought his act.
Be thou familiar, but by no means vulgar.
Those friends thou hast, and their adoption tried,
Grapple them to thy soul with hoops of steel,
But do not dull thy palm with entertainment
Of each new-hatch'd, unfledged comrade. Beware
Of entrance to a quarrel; but being in,
Bear't that the opposed may beware of thee.
Give every man thy ear, but few thy voice;
Take each man's censure, but reserve thy judgment.
Costly thy habit as thy purse can buy,
But not express'd in fancy; rich, not gaudy,
For the apparel oft proclaims the man,
And they in France of the best rank and station
Are of a most select and generous chief in that.
Neither a borrower nor a lender be;
For loan oft loses both itself and friend,
And borrowing dulls the edge of husbandry.
This above all: to thine own self be true,
And it must follow, as the night the day,
Thou canst not then be false to any man.'

Hamlet, Act I, Scene III, Polonius to Laertes

1

Leaders of the Pack

The late 19th century saw some of the great sexual thinkers and researchers of the West, men such as Freud, Jung, Reich, Kinsey, Herschfield and Kraft-Ebbing, move Western psychology forward. However, it was Masters and Johnson's pioneering work in the late 1950s that blew open people's ideas about sexuality.

Before their work scientists knew virtually nothing about what really happened during sex and how people behaved. Masters and Johnson scientifically studied the responses of healthy couples having sex and ordinary people masturbating. Nothing like this had ever been attempted before. When the book of their findings was released in 1966 the timing was unintentionally perfect. A social revolution was in the air, which was to go on to have worldwide implications.

An all-too-rarely acknowledged personal revolution for men began in the late 1960s, came into full force in the 1970s and is still continuing today. It started when men began to question the notion of a single, 'normal', masculinity.

A new language emerged around the concept of 'maleness', with men wanting to look at every way in which they could expand the concept of what it was to be male. A dialogue was started, albeit in radical circles, about the social construction of masculinity and what that meant for every aspect of a man's life. From the way they dressed, to the way they had sex, men's lives were seen as being rigid and proscribed, with men who deviated from the accepted script written off as 'anti-social' or a 'loser'.

For men, a simple act such as growing their hair from the standard back and sides to something longer became seen as a radical anti-authoritarian, even anarchic, feat. It is a good measure of how rigid ideas of masculinity were at the time that such a slight deviation from the norm provoked such furious and long-standing outrage. In fact, for well over a decade 'long-haired' became the standard mainstream insult to men who challenged society in any way.

During this time men not only grew their hair long, they wore kaftans (dresses!), opposed the military, wore flowers as a political act and challenged the wounds they believed they carried as a result of a repressive, traditional male upbringing. They sought to discard dysfunctional ideas about men and masculinity and replace them with new ideas that did not rely on old stereotypes of the 'right kind of man'.

This wasn't about making men effeminate, androgynous, or more like women, nor was it about constructing a bland, passionless sexuality. The men in this chapter were pioneers in creating new ways to conceive of male sexuality, which at the time was usually associated with sexual aggression, conquest or porn-related fantasies.

For the first time in the West, this way of thinking (begun in the 1970s) revealed the possibility of male sexuality as being playful, fun and endearing. It showed that men have deep sexual longings, not just needs, and that these have an emotional depth, which, sadly for men, is more often than not unrealised.

Also at this time freethinkers turned to the traditions and customs of the 'mystic' East, as it was then seen. Many intellectuals admired Asian societies where there was no split between the spiritual, sexual and social, and all were considered to be equally important in ensuring a person's total wellbeing. This was true for men as well as women, and the idea that men had been wounded by traditional ideas about masculinity, and could be personally healed through spirituality was a very radical view at the time.

One of the West's 'discoveries' during this fascination with the East was ancient doctrines, philosophies and practices of spirituality and sexuality. Tantric teachings, which evolved in India and spread throughout Asia, astounded Westerners with the idea that heightened sexual pleasure cannot stem from physical intercourse alone. Tantra takes a need to explore awareness and consciousness and combines it with sex, which is seen as a major element of life.

The ancient Chinese philosophy of Taoism states that the liberation of the spirit must be based on the liberation of the entire being. This spiritual liberation only takes place through the full expression and understanding of the nature of human sexuality. Sexual ecstasy is seen as a universal nourishing force. Taoism and tantra see the physical body and sexuality as tools for human transformation. In these philosophies, the body is a symbol and represents the state of our inner spiritual life and even our psychological development.

Tantric sex requires a connection on all levels, not just the Western focus on the physical; an equality of mind between partners. There was no idea that men shouldn't express certain feelings, or that any emotions were off-limits. Another radical idea was that sex could be seen as an art, just as much as painting or sculpture, and that people could study and perfect their lovemaking skills over a lifetime.

The men in this chapter were early East–West bridge builders, or controversial sexual pioneers in their field. They didn't accept traditional ideas about male sexuality, challenged themselves and others, and started trends that have gone on to become worldwide movements. They saw what human sexuality could be, not just what it was, rejected outmoded concepts of masculinity and forged a radical new vision of maleness.

Joseph Kramer

Joseph Kramer grew up near the Mississippi river in the American Midwest, and comes from a religious Roman Catholic family. After spending four years training with the Jesuits he took his vows, but after 11 years he decided that his spirituality included his body and eroticism. As this was incompatible with being a Jesuit, he left the order.

In 1979 he finished a Master's degree in Erotic Spirituality from the Graduate Theological Union in Berkeley, California and completed further study in massage and breath techniques.

In 1984 he founded the Body Electric School of Massage and Rebirthing in Oakland, California. In the early years of the AIDS crisis he helped set up the first hospice massage team in the US and developed Taoist Erotic Massage. He also established the EroSpirit Research Institute in 1992, which explores all aspects of sexual growth. Since this time he has created and taught dozens of erotic rituals to thousands of men and women in the US and Europe, produced over 20 educational videos and has written extensively on erotic touch.

At present he is finishing a doctorate at the Institute for the Advanced Study of Human Sexuality. Joseph's Web site addresses are: www.erospirit.org and www.eroticmassage.com.

I started to explore sex in 1976 and decided that this was my area of interest, not from an academic perspective, but from a practical, experimental experience. For four years my passion for sex led me into all sorts of sexual interaction, often for hours and hours and hours a day. I learnt that touch was very important for good sex and that I was deficient in touching skills. In 1979 I started my study of various Californian touch therapies, including movement and body massage courses. I was seduced by Jane Fonda's aerobics classes and continued doing aerobics every day for five years.

After I had finished my Master's degree in Erotic Spirituality at the Graduate Theological Union in Berkeley, I secured an internship in counselling at the University of California in Berkeley, working mainly with gay male students. I wanted to teach a touch class but I was told this was not allowed for counsellors. So I decided to leave counselling, because I felt it was so limiting, and even now, though I have a Master's degree, and have been trained in counselling techniques for sexual minorities, I never use this training formally.

At that time the massage I had studied was called 'clinical touch', which means that the interactions with the client had nothing to do with sex. Although I knew touch and sex were all intertwined, I followed the dictates of the massage establishment and did not do any sexual erotic work on my clients. I even remember being offended by gay male clients asking me to massage their genitals.

I decided to take my massage skills further and in 1980 I trained for a year with Claire Arneson in breathwork. The programme I did with her included instruction in the rebirthing breath (with more emphasis on the inhale than the exhale), while masturbating and visualising various scenes from my past. Some of Claire's exercises to dispel shame included visualising my mother and father watching me masturbate while saying, 'We love you and we love every aspect of you.'

This was not about sex with parents, the Oedipal aspect, but just allowing them to witness me and accept me, and alerted me to the importance of 'witnessing' as a negative or positive influence. Another exercise I did was to imagine myself masturbating on the church altar of my youth. While breathing I imagined the priest, the congregation and, most importantly, God watching me, saying, 'How wonderful.' This was very helpful in clearing out negative sexual spiritual connections, the feelings of shame, guilt and sin.

This training and guidance was the beginning of me experiencing the joy of my sexuality. In 1982 I decided to open a school for touch, breathwork and erotic expression, but it took two years of preparation, finding money, teachers and creating a clearer vision. In 1984 I started the Body Electric School in Oakland, California. Initially I taught about sexuality in lecture form because I was afraid of being erotic. But at the same time AIDS was devastating the gay male community of the San Francisco Bay area.

We knew it was a disease that was sexually transmitted but we did not know much more than that. Many people shut down sexually, while others were sick and dying. There was an enormous need among the gay male community for healing and this focused my teaching. In 1983 and 1984 I developed Taoist Erotic Massage, a no-risk way of sexually relating to another.

This massage involved intense genital stimulation, while the receiver consciously breathed fast and deep. It allayed many men's fears in the AIDS era because it included erotic touch but no bodily fluids and no ejaculation. Initially I did this massage individually and then started teaching. Eventually I sent teachers throughout America, Europe, New Zealand and Australia.

The main focus with these trainings was breath, eye contact, erotic touch and no shame. The first years of erotic massage classes were only for men, but then I developed with my friend Annie Sprinkle Taoist Erotic Massage for women. For me the erotic is best experienced not as a short but intense climax but as a prolonged, creative, transformative state.

TIPS: To help you experience more pleasure

Often when people try to experience more pleasure they will hear many voices from their past, condemning them. I call these witnesses and judges. These voices may be from your parents, teachers, priests or peers, people who have shamed you with their words and actions. The major way I have found to change this insidious pattern is to breath consciously when in sexual situations. This keeps you in the present moment and disengages the negative messages from the past. I have learnt various breathing techniques from rebirthing, Taoism, tantra and Sufi practices.

If a couple is breathing together as they make love then they are present to one another. You can immediately tell if your partner becomes distracted because his or her breathing changes. Playing with various breathing rhythms is central to love play and pleasure.

EXERCISE: MASTURBATING MOMENTS TO ENHANCE SEX FOR MEN OR WOMEN

Using a video camera, film yourself masturbating. This exercise will give you biofeedback about how you move your body, how fully you breathe and how consciously you touch yourself as you masturbate. The result is not to have yourself starring in a porn video. Masturbate as you usually do; do not act or play to the camera. The video you take will allow you to see how you are with your body. You will see what your sexual partner sees, your constrictions and your enjoyment.

Over a two-week period video yourself five times masturbating. You must set up the camera so you can see your total body and include sound. This exercise can take from three minutes to 20 minutes or more. The length of your solo lovemaking doesn't matter. Immediately after you have finished taping yourself, watch the video with a notebook. Write down what you observe in the video. Often, in the first session, many people are shocked because they don't look as if they are enjoying themselves.

Look carefully at your body. Do you see tension and where? Be aware of your breathing and the sound you are making. Is this a joyous experience, a celebration of self? Stop the video and write down all your observations. Note also your feelings as you watch yourself. This information will help you to change and develop what is not working for you.

I have found that 90 per cent of what people write down is negative. They are surprised to see how stressful this experience is.

When you do your second video session, be sure not to perform for the camera. Perform for yourself. Again, watch the results and take notes. Compare the sessions to see if you are more relaxed. Are you still embarrassed while watching yourself or is there a bit more acceptance? Continue this taping for another three sessions.

It takes a lot of discipline and commitment to do this exercise, but I have never had a person who has completed this process who has not felt it was one of the most transformative sexual experiences of his or her life. By the end of five sessions you will know what you want to change and what you like and accept about yourself. Often women comment on how much they enjoyed the depth of their sexuality, and how sometimes they felt distracted from their own sexuality during sex with their partner. Almost all persons who do this exercise learn to have more enjoyment while masturbating.

Watching yourself is a great educational tool because for many people masturbation is based on shame and the idea that this is second-rate sexuality. Masturbation is a way for you to touch and enjoy your body, and I feel that this is a sensual ritual that children should learn to do. Harley Swiftdeer, an American Indian shaman, teaches that masturbation is 'heart pleasuring'. In other words, as you masturbate, you open up your heart and your capacity to love. This correlates with the Taoist teaching that sexual energy, or 'Ching Chi', becomes compassion when circulated through the heart.

Our sexuality often falters because we have no connection to ourself. We look outside ourself for someone to love us. This creates many problems in relationships because there is the feeling that my sexuality is nothing without a partner.

What a powerful exercise it can be to masturbate in front of your partner. If you feel your partner is not judging or ridiculing you but looking at you in wonderment, then shame is banished.

I have found that the resources we need to help us learn erotic touch are not readily available. So I founded The New School of Erotic Touch, with a Web site that offers the finest video classes in erotic touch available in the world. My staff and I have previewed over 200 videos and the best are available at www.eroticmassage.com.

You cannot learn touch by watching these videos. You can only learn by actually practising the touch along with the video demonstrations. So get your remote control into a plastic baggie and start learning some new ways to touch yourself and others.

Mantak Chia

Mantak Chia is famous for his books on cultivating male and female sexuality, and for founding a system known as The Healing Tao, now known as The Universal Tao. Today he has over 1,000 certified instructors, and thousands of practitioners, throughout the world who are teaching and practising the Taoist arts, from healing to t'ai chi, and offering benefits ranging from stress relief to longevity.

He was born in 1944 in Bangkok to Chinese parents. His grandfather was a Baptist minister, the first break in many generations of Taoist healers, and as a young boy, in a land of Buddhism, with strong Hindu and animist influences, he found himself brought up as a Christian.

He studied with Taoist and Buddhist masters in meditation, aikido, yoga, t'ai chi, Thai boxing, kung fu and other esoteric practices. He also studied Western medicine and anatomy for two years. In his centres in the USA, Canada, Europe and Thailand and in his many books, The Multi-orgasmic Man, Awaken Healing Energy Through the Tao, Taoist Secrets of Love: Cultivating Male Sexual Energy *and* Healing Love Through the Tao: Cultivating Female Sexual Energy, *he teaches the Taoist ways to transform stress into vitality.*

He has taught men and women Iron Shirt Chi Kung and Fusion of the Five Elements. These ancient Chinese Taoist techniques link sexual energy and transcendent states of consciousness. After 20 years in the West, he now lives and works at the Tao Garden in Chiang Mai in northern Thailand, in the home and healing meditation centre he has created.

The West lacks the essence of the spiritual practice and real experience of it, as it has more emphasis on the material world. People are dependent on priests, physiologists and therapy for their emotional health, rather than themselves. With sexuality and spirituality, they do not understand much about good physical sex and how to use sexual energy for healing. It is important that people understand what the Tao principle is, as it sets people free from physical sickness and emotional dependence and spiritual dependence.

I make my life's work teaching about spiritual sexuality. I have practised my theories, and I can see the result in the spiritual and sexual practices for healing and increasing the brainpower. Sexual energy is the basic energy for the body. It is the building block for the body and brain.

The traditional Taoist masters taught one-on-one, never to foreigners, and closely guarded their ancient secrets. However, I have written 12 books and taught Westerners in a very Western way, with workshops and group seminars. This came about because my teacher, the hermit White Cloud, was the last of the long lineage of masters from Long White Mountain at Chang Bai San near Manchuria.

Seeing the traditional way of the Tao being repressed in his homeland, he feared the secrets of long life and good health would be lost. In exile in Hong Kong, he saw how other masters charged too much money for these secrets, just giving to one or two pupils. He felt the way to keep the Taoist practices alive was to bring them into modern society so that many could benefit. He instructed me to teach Westerners, but first to prove my roots with my own people.

I taught first in my home city of Bangkok and then in the Chinese community in New York. My main work was healing and Taoist spiritual work, but it was the sexual practices that caught the attention of Western students. These secret arts were originally taught to enable an emperor to enjoy his harem of wives and concubines without depleting his energies. Although I was brought up a Christian, I didn't accept the Christian idea of sex as sin because sexual practices are healing practices, healing the self, healing relationships.

It is only sin if you see it as sin. Sex is natural, not sinful. The human being has a powerful sex drive – and you cannot keep ping-pong balls under water. Sometime, somewhere, they pop back up, maybe as disease, maybe as emotional problems, causing energy blockages, leading to illness.

Sex is your servant, not your master. Who am I to decide where and when, or whom you do it with? This is between you and your conscience. I teach how to control and harness the sexual energy, energy powerful enough for a man to repopulate a continent with a single ejaculation. And every woman is born with enough eggs to generate hundreds of lives. Without reproduction all that power is wasted. If we are not using the hormones and nutrients of sexual activity to start a new life we can recycle it to make our own life longer, healthier, more enjoyable. Not repressing, recycling!

All systems make moral statements, but they all say different things. Some religions say sex with corpses is a sacred path to enlightenment, with others you may have several wives at once, while in others you go to hell for an impure thought. What is impure thought? Every man secretly imagines being an emperor, having many women, even monks, priests and even saints. Saint Augustine said, 'Lord, give me chastity, but please, not just yet.'

Some systems try to make us feel guilty for thinking natural thoughts. Yet these urges make our human species so successful, so strong, to survive so many generations. Imagine an enlightened being descending to earth now and telling us it is sinful to move our bowels. We cannot help moving our bowels, it is a natural function. So is sex. In the Tao we say, No right or wrong, no good or bad, just recycling the energy.

I still consider myself a Christian, but I don't belong to any church, although I may start one here in the Tao Garden – we have already married three couples. The churches teach about it being bad to do this, bad to do that. We don't have to be taught what's bad: it comes naturally. Or doing what comes naturally – they call it bad!

The Western God is dominant male, very yang, enforcing laws with fear of punishment, saying you will burn in hell. Society reflects this, with laws enforced by violence. Now there is imbalance between the yang of justice and the yin of compassion. True religion is about love and compassion. You can be Hindu, Jewish, Buddhist or Muslim and still enjoy the benefits of Tao in the framework of your own belief system.

I have written a book [called] *Multi-orgasmic Man*, but it is women who are naturally multi-orgasmic. One of my earliest books was about healing through the Tao [and] cultivating female sexual energy. Woman is considered yin. Yang and yin cannot exist without each other, so it is better if they are in harmony. Taoist practice promotes harmony, because when the man, considered yang, lets go of semen, he is drained, but the woman is ready for more. When both are in tune, they have increased vigour, improved stamina, enhanced sensation and unlimited whole-body orgasms. The ideal is the multi-orgasmic couple and the Taoist sexual practices are self-healing for couples.

Conserving energy by seminal retention is an exclusively male practice, but women can also obtain the benefits of health and longevity. Although women do not normally lose too much energy through orgasm, they do through menstruation and childbirth. Taoist practices for women recycle menstrual energy, with the same benefits of long life, good health and painless menstruation.

For man, seminal retention by itself is not enough; non-ejaculatory orgasm without opening the Microcosmic Orbit leads to blockages in the sexual centre, sometimes with aching limbs, congestion, wet dreams and headaches. Both man and woman must redirect their energy through the Microcosmic Orbit, what the classics call the Small Heavenly Cycle. As above, so below – within each one of us is also a small universe, a small cosmos, yin and yang flowing together. In the act of sex, the moment of orgasm, yin and yang unite and the two heavenly cycles become one. Including these techniques in your lovemaking, with yourself or a partner, is the key to making sex a spiritual experience.

The Microcosmic Orbits are the two major channels in acupuncture known as functional and governor channels. Usually we start by concentrating in the navel area, feeling it become warm and starting to spiral, in a counter-clockwise direction in a horizontal way, till chi pressure builds up. We use the mind to guide the chi to flow down to the perineum and down to leg bones and feel the chi in the bones.

You can then develop your practice further and extend it to the Macrocosmic Orbit, so the sexual energy can transfer up to the crown and extend to the cosmos and combine into the cosmic orgasm, which is the major sexual spiritual practice.

The Microcosmic Orbit, as I first described it many years ago, has since appeared in books by various Westerners on love, sex, tantra, sex-magic and shamanism. I'm glad they like it, and if it helps people to more fulfilled lives, they are helping me and I am grateful, and happy to help them. But some techniques can be dangerous if not done with care and preparation. For example, I am teaching Taoist tantra, which has common roots with Hindu and Buddhist Kundalini practices.

The Taoist way puts safety first, working with the energy-body, making sure channels are open and clear at each stage before going on to the next. We also practice t'ai chi and Iron Shirt Chi Kung to keep grounded. With some Indo/Tibetan (Hindu/Buddhist) systems there can be the danger of activating too much energy before clearing channels and without proper grounding. This can overload the nervous system, with many painful side effects. Tantra is known as the short path to enlightenment, but this short path could actually mean one whole lifetime of preparation and practice. You cannot learn it in a weekend.

The Taoist Canons describe how a group of Aryans were shipwrecked on the South China shore thousands of years ago. They did not die, or have children, and became known as the Shining Ones. They transmitted their secret magical and healing practices to the shamans. When Buddhism came to China, shamans were persecuted, like witches in the West, so they became Taoists, rivals to the Buddhists, and continued their practices in secret, using only internal energy, internal alchemy, without the use of accessories to identify themselves. The saying goes you cannot tell a sage by his clothes. They were also known as magicians, wizards and sorcerers. Yes, Taoism is magic.

It is unknown what happened to the Shining Ones. Maybe they are still around, but not in their physical body. They could leave when they want, astral travel, and come back when they want. Magic is like religion. It can be of great benefit, or cause great harm. In Taoist magic as in the Tao, there is no judgement – we are all responsible for ourselves. As long as you do not harm another being, you are free to do what you want.

I am a high-tech Taoist. I use mobile phones, computers and watch television. I think technology is very good when it releases us from drudgery. With electronics, you can keep yourself safe from electronic pollution inside an energy bubble, by creating an insulating bubble around the equipment. As you know from our Taoist healing practices, you can seal yourself from the condition of your patients, even serious contagious diseases.

The cosmic healing practice is to internalise disease, then cleanse, energise and restore healthy energy to the patient. Energy is vibration, and if we get the vibration right, nothing bad gets through. This is psychic self-defence, very important for healers. The more you work with contaminated energy, the more you need the protective practices, from Inner Smile right through to Kan & Li. This gives external protection, internal clarity and helps us live in modern society, and use the technology available without causing damage to ourselves.

My teaching has changed over the years, become less formulaic, more intuitive. The old masters taught one-to-one, reciting secret formulas obscured in codes. Many people could not read or write in those days. They just practised the formulas, learning by experience and repetition, not asking questions, trusting the master. That is how I learnt from White Cloud, and how I started teaching. Now I've taught in the West for over 20 years, with workshops and group seminars.

Westerners have intellectual appreciation for theory. I have the benefit of feedback from my own direct students and over 1,000 Universal Tao instructors and their students. So we evolve and adapt. I learn from my students. The material is the same, just the delivery changes. Interpretation also changes, as modern science tells us things about the energy field that ancient Taoists knew but did not have the vocabulary to explain and anyway wanted to keep secret. Now, for example, Deepak Chopra is investigating ageing, talks about energy information, energy intelligence, bioelectromagnetic force. This is a modern scientist giving real sense of the meaning to what he calls 'Prana', and the Taoist classics call 'Qi'.

What is immortality? Keeping the same body forever, or awareness of your spirit in different incarnations? What is important is to be present in this life, learn to transform stress into vitality, develop compassion through love, recycle energy to keep the body healthy and in harmony with mind and spirit, learn to understand true nature as spirit. Then you are open to possibilities beyond the cycle of life and death.

If a sage died many hundreds of years old, then he is dead, not immortal! White Cloud told me his teacher was 250 years old. He had to go to his cave and put wax in the teacher's nose and other orifices to keep out insects and dust, and make sure the body was not eaten while his teacher's spirit was away travelling to source.

Stan Dale

Dr Stan Dale is a transactional analyst, educator, workshop facilitator and author. A New Yorker by birth, he spent 19 years in Chicago, where he originated and hosted the first psychologically based radio call-in talk show in the US. Prior to that he was the announcer/narrator for The Lone Ranger, Sergeant Preston of the Yukon *and* The Green Hornet, *and for a brief period was the voice of The Shadow on radio.*

For more than 20 years after his arrival in San Francisco, Stan was the host of numerous radio talk shows and continues to be in constant demand on television shows including Donahue, Oprah, Joan Rivers, Geraldo, CNBC, Sally Jessy Raphael *and many more too numerous to mention.*

He has written two books, Fantasies Can Set You Free *and* My Child, My Self: How to Raise the Child You Always Wanted to Be, *and he is featured in the best-selling books* Chicken Soup for the Soul, Bridges to Heaven *and many others.*

Dr Dale has advanced degrees in psychology and sociology from Roosevelt University, Chicago and the Illinois Institute of Applied Psychology. He received his Doctorate in Human Sexuality from The Institute for the Advanced Study of Human Sexuality in San Francisco, where he is Adjunct Professor of Behavioural Studies in Human Sexuality.

Dr Dale has been on the faculties of Loyola University, Mundelein College in Chicago and Sonoma State University in Cotati, California. He is a frequent lecturer at many colleges and universities in California and elsewhere, including China's Shandong and Beijing universities, where he is a visiting professor. Dr Dale speaks to a wide variety of service and civic organisations, social clubs, churches, high school and junior high school campuses as well as corporations.

After serving with the US Army in Korea, he received a commendation and Ribbon of Meritorious Service. He is one of only 10 worldwide recipients of the prized Mahatma Gandhi Peace Medallion, for his selfless commitment to the cause of world peace, humanity and brotherhood. He was also presented with the Humanitarian of the Year award from the Ethical Humanists of Chicago and has received the Distinguished Member Award of Who's Who Worldwide.

In 1968, Dr Dale created The Human Awareness Institute. Since then more than 50,000 people have attended the Institute's workshops and seminars in various parts of the US, Russia, Europe, Australia and Japan.

I always feel humble that I was considered one of 10 people to receive the Mahatma Gandhi Peace Medallion. I tried giving it away to people who I felt deserved it more but they refused to accept it. It was given to me for the work I did during the Vietnam war. I went to the Paris peace conference and did my part on radio and television to end the war and to help bring some sanity back to the planet.

I feel that I have been drawn to the work I have done through the pain and suffering I have gone through in my life. It is not worse than anyone else's, but it came about specifically when I was drafted into the military and having my two children taken away from me. There was a lot of bitterness between my wife [and I] at that time, which had been going on and on. Its basis was that she wanted me to accept Christ as my personal saviour, as she had become a born-again Christian. I said that was wonderful and that I supported her in this, but she wanted me and the children to accept Christ.

I said that you couldn't do it that way – we have to come to that decision by ourselves. She could not accept that and said that if I can't have you, and Christ can't have you, then the army will have you. She had me drafted because there was a paragraph in our draft laws that stated that if your marital status in any way changed you would lose your deferment. I had been deferred because I had two children prior to the Korean War.

I had been a well-known radio personality called 'The Voice of The Shadow' and 'The Lone Ranger', both of which were very popular. At the time I was drafted I felt like my whole life had been destroyed.

However, in the topsy-turvy way that the world works there was a motion picture being filmed in a geisha house outside Tokyo. At that time I was in the armed forces radio and television service, and I was asked to a cast party there, and that was where my real adventure began. My whole world was turned upside down.

In 1957 I was invited to live at the geisha house for seven months and there I found my heart, soul and life purpose. I learnt about reverence, divinity and compassion; there was nothing about sex in the geisha house. I was trained in a way that I would never have expected. It was in the simple things like looking at a flower, looking at a human being and seeing the magnificence in everything. If God wanted to hide, he would hide in human beings because it was the last place human beings would think to look, and this approach opened new worlds for me. I was then able to see the god and goddess in each person. This belief has only got stronger and stronger for me since this time.

I had always thought I was going to be a radio announcer for the rest of my life. I had no intention of starting The Human Awareness Institute [HAI]. Interestingly, 'Hai' means 'yes' in Japanese and 'life' in Hebrew, and 'the sea' in Chinese, as in Chang Hai, the city by the sea. When I came back to the US from Japan I went back into radio and was bored, but used this time to finish degrees in sociology and psychology.

In 1968, during my regular five-hour nightly radio programme people would ring in to talk to me about life, sexuality and other things but none of that would go to air. I went to management to see if I could put some of these calls to air. Initially they were very hesitant and I was told to make them short, quick and then play records. At the end of two weeks we were averaging 100,000 people per night ringing in from all over the US. There had been nothing like this in the world before and everyone was astounded that people needed and wanted to talk so publicly. Finally it became a talkback radio programme where people could ring up and talk about everything, and through this I started the HAI.

People were asking for more, as they wanted to get together, so in 1968 I rented a hall and 1,500 people showed up for a 'love-in' with Stan Dale. People spent the day asking questions and this became the basis of the Human Awareness Institute.

A Japanese woman working in Tokyo came to Chicago to do the workshop and she loved it so much she organised workshops in Japan, and from this basis the workshops have spread all over the world.

The basic tenets of the workshops are respect, dignity, compassion, love, understanding and trust. All of that is what every human being on the planet hungers for.

Most people in our culture haven't the foggiest idea what sex is. If I were to ask anyone where did they learn about sex, outside workshops we learn it catch-as-catch-can. How do you know what you are learning is not absolute garbage? I am a Doctor of Human Sexuality and I know most people have no real understanding of sex. They think it's intercourse, they think it concerns the genitals, but sex is not this at all. It is really about sacred energy exchange, spiritual energy exchange, sensual energy exchange, every human being has energy and can exchange it with another.

When my energy touches your energy it is an energy exchange. How do we do that? Is it through the genitals, or do I look at you, or hold you, or breathe with you? The average human body is 3,500 square inches of skin – that doesn't include the mind, the heart and the soul. Most people see sex like a fast food diet, when they could be having a delicious banquet of 35 hundred square inches. Where are you going to learn that? We are always going through different stages of maturation and awareness and our senses have not been revered enough.

When you look at a sunrise and your body starts to shiver through the beauty of it, these are little orgasms. When someone touches you and strokes your arm, or back, or hair and your body starts to shudder, these are orgasms. We are so poor in our culture because what we think about sex is so limited, there is so much more. I can get deeper into my partner with my eyes than with any part of my body. I see people who have taken our courses open to their sexuality as if they were seeing a huge sunrise instead of a sliver of light. What is love, what is sexuality, unfortunately many people are only in the early stages of learning.

Most people don't have a good body image. The advertisers have done a great job in making us believe we are either too fat, too old, too much grey hair, our teeth and eyes are never quite right. What can the advertisers sell you if you think you are beautiful? But if you think you are ugly then they can sell you anything and everything.

If you don't believe you are beautiful, yet you want me to be in a relationship with you, what are you offering me? You want me to love and accept you. You want me to think you are beautiful, but if I do then you think there is something wrong with me. People have never seen their real body – when they look in the mirror they see the reverse. Human beings have never really seen themselves.

EXERCISE: CREATING A POSITIVE MENTAL FANTASY

Why do you think negatively about any part of yourself?

As an adult your job is to say thank you very much for your early input from your parents, teachers and others, which no longer applies to you. Say to yourself, 'As an adult I am a magnificent human being.'

You will never hear a tree say, 'I am ugly' or 'My branches aren't quite right', or 'If only my leaves were a different colour'. Nothing in nature other than humans tell themselves that they are not OK. When you compare yourself you are only comparing yourself to other human beings who have never seen themselves. It's a paradox; we have been programmed just like computers.

If you are having difficulty believing this you can make yourself a tape. Have someone you care about say to you, 'You are a beautiful man/woman just the way you are, a unique work of art on the planet.' The biggest lie you were told was that if you loved yourself you would be self-centred and egotistical, but it's actually the opposite. If you don't love yourself you will act egotistically, and be self-centred and narcissistic.

2

Sexual Spirit

In the area of sexual performance it is usually women who have grabbed the publicity and the headlines. Men have had the gaze, and women have been the performers. While male performance artists have done spectacular work, often it has not encompassed sex, or been sexually challenging. Many people are still surprised to hear of a male artist using sexual performance as his medium, and as a vehicle for his artistic growth.

When 'male' and 'sexual' and 'performance' appear in the same sentence most people's response is to immediately think of a troupe of male strippers such as The Chippendales, or to remember with a laugh films such as *The Full Monty*.

The men in this chapter have been and are extraordinary and exceptional performance artists. They have created new rituals around the body and sexuality, seen performance and indeed sex itself as an art form and used their creative talents to be open to the magic of sex. They have seen the world in a different way and sought to express this publicly.

Sexuality has traditionally been seen as private and the idea that sexual energy can be channelled into creativity makes many people uncomfortable. However, the men profiled have often expressed themselves joyously, which has won them some unlikely converts. Some take on the persona of a court jester; others are more in-your-face, taking people out of their comfort zone, to the edge, and pushing them over so they can fly.

Ritual performance goes back to the earliest human records and was used for creative as well as social purposes. It also allows for taboo subjects to be broached and dealt with: demons may be conjured up by a ritual, but they are defeated and banished as well.

Sexual performance artists believe that the repression of sexuality, one of the most essential human needs, has caused it to be expressed in ways that are unhealthy and even toxic. One of these is the rigid gender roles that assign universal human qualities as either exclusively male or female.

The most exciting performance artists are using sex to challenge the balance between masculine and feminine energies. They argue that if one part of your self is internalised, because certain emotions are not deemed as belonging to your biological gender, then they probably need expression in some part of your life. As men have been trained to be dominant, competitive and aggressive, so radical male performance artists have made the opposite the basis of their sexual explorations. They have often taken on expressions of submissiveness (long seen as archetypically female), frequently by vulnerably exposing the body in a public place. Experiments with sexual healing have involved pagan-inspired sex with trees, and blatantly subverting the male sexual gaze and turning it towards other men.

At the height of the AIDS hysteria in the US in the 1980s performance artists challenged taboos about body fluids in confrontationalist performances. Their hardcore rituals saw them rawly exposed to other human bodies at a time when there was a fever pitch of emotion about any un-latexed human contact.

Their work is characterised by not seeing limitations, only possibilities, as they strip back maleness and sexuality to its (often literally) bare essentials. It is a courageous act in a society that, for all its talk of gender-bending, still punishes the man who steps out of his assigned gender role. They see their work as not just personally and artistically challenging for themselves, but as a vehicle for enriching the world and changing rigid old ideas of gender and sexuality. They are doing the work described by philosopher J. Krishnamurti in *The First and Last Freedom*, when he says:

> To transform the world we must begin with ourselves: and what is important in the beginning with ourselves is the intention… this is our responsibility, yours and mine; because however small may be the world we live in, if we can bring about a radically different point of view in our daily existence then perhaps we shall affect the world at large.

Willem de Ridder

Willem de Ridder was born in the Netherlands. He grew up as a magician, puppeteer, storyteller and performer. He used these skills in his first radio plays, made on his dad's home-made tape recorder, long before these machines were for sale. His artistic talent led him to study at the Academy for Art and Design in 's-Hertogenbosch. In the 1960s de Ridder used music as a creative medium in the areas of fashion, ballet, theatre and art, co-founding the Mood Engineering Society. This led him to organise concerts and Flux performance festivals. He then became chairman for Fluxus in Northern Europe, running the first Fluxus mail order warehouse.

He designed SUCK, *the first European sex newspaper, which had a cult following worldwide and led to the first erotic film festival in the world. After moving to Hollywood he started Radio Cadillac and continued with the production of sex magazines. This unfortunately proved so controversial that the federal police became involved and de Ridder moved to Italy to publish* Hate and Love *for the American market.*

Through radio, theatre and magazines in Europe and the US he continued to explore his storytelling. In Rhode Island he was arrested with Annie Sprinkle for producing pornography. This led to a romance with her and a return to Italy to work on organising visual arts concerts and avant-garde theatre, as well as using his talents with music and stories in radio and television.

He presented The Sprinkle Salon *on NY cable and directed Annie Sprinkle's one-woman show* Postporn Modernist*, which has played throughout the world. He co-founded the New Ancient Sex Academy with Cora Emens, which focuses on a spiritual approach to sexuality. De Ridder now has weekly talk shows on Amsterdam TV and radio and continues to give his workshops and seminars on mirrorology, as well as working with the corporate sector. You can listen and chat to him every Friday on www.willemderidder.com.*

One of the things that has always intrigued me about sexuality is that you have to start at the very beginning. Most men seem to get no sexual instruction whatsoever. I learnt about sex on the streets and did not get a very good picture of it. I quickly found out that there were many people around who also had received little sex instruction. This inspired me years later to start a newspaper in Amsterdam for the 60s generation called *Hitweek*, which was completely written by the readers. Whatever they wrote, as well as photographs, were unedited and ran uncensored.

People from all ages started to write about all different topics. At the beginning it was mostly about music but over time it became more and more sexual. For the time this was really outspoken. More and more people in their late teens and early twenties became regular contributors and out of this came a new generation of scriptwriters, journalists and artists because previously there had been no medium for them to express themselves.

Hitweek became world famous and I was contacted by people in England to set up a national newspaper for them about sexuality, which would have been illegal for them to do there. We started the paper and it included the editor of *The International Times* in the UK, William Levy, Heathcote Williams, who is a very famous poet now, Jim Haynes, who ran the Arts Laboratory, Jean Shrimpton the model and Germaine Greer the feminist.

We called the newspaper *SUCK*, and after the first issue the UK police came, but there was very little they could do because we were in Holland. We organised the first pornographic film festival in the world, which was very political, with artists and intellectuals from all over the world coming together.

Through this time I met all sorts of people, and I had relationships and sex, but didn't think very much about it other than that something was missing. I started talking to people about it and read about Taoism, which had been translated by intellectuals, and they all wrote about Chinese Taoist men that had the possibility of not ejaculating, but shooting their sperm up their spine. At the time I thought this was ridiculous.

During this period I had set up clubs like Paradiso and Fantasio in Amsterdam, where the audience performed their own programme with acts, happenings, dancing and music. Soon there were about 150 clubs like that all over the country. Sex soon became a major theme and I realised there was a great need for a school where people could learn more about sex. I thought that sex should be open, talked about and studied seriously beyond 'wham, bam, thank you ma'am'. When I proposed it, everybody was shocked. It was too early for an academy of advanced sexuality... in puritanical Holland.

I went to Los Angeles. It was in the early 1970s and I studied macrobiotics, shiatsu and Chinese medicine in Hollywood. One day I found a newspaper that had been reconstructed from *SUCK*. I soon found out that Maximilian Lobckovicz (an Italian/Czechoslovakian prince) was behind it. He and I banded together and started a similar newspaper called *FINGER* and soon contributions came in by the ton. I quickly found out that America was even more puritanical than Europe at that time.

Every week there was a bust by the police because none of the contributions were censored. The letters I received became more outspoken and unusual, from topics of incest, amputation and mutilation to faecal fetishes. Through this I started a new magazine called *GOD*, with stories that were so unbelievable that the printer freaked out and I had to call it *G:The magazine with the secret name*. Nevertheless *G* sold out in three hours. I started to get death threats, so after a few issues my staff got scared. These magazines were distributed through the sex shops and had a big influence on *Playboy* and *Penthouse*. *Hustler* was totally inspired by us.

Maximilian and I had to escape to Europe and continued producing our magazines from there. They became more and more popular in America. Through this I was asked to return to the States to produce a magazine for Annie Sprinkle, who was a famous porn star in New York. Our typesetter turned out to be an undercover agent and we were arrested. The media went berserk and Annie and I decided to live together in Italy for a year.

When I came back to Amsterdam I started a relationship with Cora Emens and we opened a school called the New Ancient Sex Academy, running workshops, bringing Joseph Kramer out from the US to teach body massage and body energy. Suddenly I started to understand the Taoist writings I had originally read, realising it was all about sexual energy or chi. This led to me researching my own sexual energy. I found a lesbian massagist who was very interested too. Every week we practised for about eight hours a new type of masturbation.

When we normally masturbate, we mostly tense all our muscles, closing off all our energy channels. We pump up the energy in the genital area, where it is stuck. It's like blowing up a balloon. Soon we explode, we lose all energy and fall asleep. We call that orgasm. We tried to relax instead of being sexually excited, which creates tension, which closes our energy channels. Through massage and breathing we explored sexual energy and after months of persevering I was able to experience a deep inner silence with pulsing energy orgasms, without even touching my genitals.

I hadn't seen Annie Sprinkle for some time, and when I started directing her sexual performance show I found that she had also been exploring her spiritual–sexual energy and she had experienced similar things herself. This inspired me to run workshops with couples to help them expand their erotic energy. Since I started to experience this depth of sexual energy, I can make love for hours without ejaculating. This is not just important in the area of sexuality, but in all areas of your life and creativity.

Exercise: Tips for expanding your sexual energy

Don't force your sexual energy. It doesn't work. Anything that you put energy into grows, so if you force then the forcing will grow. Don't focus on orgasms or the outcome.

If you try to comfort your partner, you lose yourself. If you touch your partner, you are feeling only your own body. So you can only make it very pleasurable for yourself. If you feel great, your partner will feel great too. We're ONE. Relax your body and thoughts. By breathing deeply and rhythmically you are able to be present with your own sensations.

To expand and give yourself pleasure, move your body and make sounds. Even if you act as if you experience great pleasure, your body will follow.

Watch obsessive sexual fantasising. By having sexual fantasies all your sexual energy goes into them instead of in your body.

If there are 10 parts of pleasure that can be reached woman is able to reach all 10, while a man has access to about four. The most pleasure a man gets is when the woman reaches orgasm; a man is a sexual servant to the woman. So it is very important that he is able to control his ejaculation, by being totally relaxed instead of excited.

A woman sends out sexual energy, which grows up to the time she menstruates. All men are strongly affected by that energy. If a man doesn't give loving attention to his partner around the period of menstruation, she will get furious, mean and sometimes violent and unfortunately most men don't understand why.

Keith Hennessy

*Keith Hennessy is a Canadian-born, interdisciplinary artist and community organiser living in San Francisco. His award-winning solo performances (*Saliva, Sacred Boy, The King is Dead, Heat, Ecstatic Songs & Manifestos, Box, Palpitations*) have been produced at gay and lesbian festivals in Sydney, Los Angeles, Seattle, Toronto and Auckland, and at theatres across the US. Currently Hennessy tours with Cahin-Caha,* cirque bâtard, *an international team of mongrel circus artists based in France. From 1985–94 he was a principal collaborator in CONTRABAND, an award-winning, internationally acclaimed performance company.*

From 1994–98 he trained and performed with CORE, a collective of multi-disciplinary artists. In 1995 he received significant commissions from the Jerome Foundation and the Walker Art Center for Unsafe, Unsuited *with Patrick Scully and Ishmael Houston-Jones, and the SF Art Commission's Market St Art in Transit Program for* The Blue Family *with K. Ruby. In 1997, Keith won the Bay Area Theater Critics Award for Best Choreography for the historic remake of* Crimes Against Nature. *In 1999 Keith won two Izzy awards (with partners Curtis and Beckman) for* Ice Car Cage.

Hennessy is co-director of 848 Community Space, a thriving urban site for cultural experiments and recipient of the 1996 SF Focus/Stolichnaya Arts Achievement Award. It hosts ongoing rituals, workshops and sex parties dedicated to the sexual liberation of all.

In the nineties Keith taught performance at New College of California, directed original performance works by students at Redwood and San Andreas high schools, and led sex and intimacy rituals for Body Electric School. Hennessy has worked as a consultant and curator and is a member of Alternate ROOTS, a visionary service organisation for community-based artists. He co-edited the book More Out Than In: Notes on Sex, Art & Community, *and his essays have been published in the magazines* Contact Quarterly, Changing Men, Movement Research *and* RFD.

With Joseph Kramer and John Pasqualetti he developed Body Electric's Sacred Intimate training for male sexual healers. With Jack Davis he created Phallic/Image, a series of pagan sex rituals and nude workshops for queer men, including HomoHex, an annual naked ritual and street spectacle.

*Hennessy has presided at all of Body Electric's large-scale rituals (*Touch NYC, [Washington] DC, SF [San Francisco]*), facilitating up to 150 men in ecstatic rites of intimacy and pleasure. Hennessy has been a friend and consultant to scores of male and female sex workers.*

When the words 'I am a sexual healer' first came through my body and out my mouth I cried, the release was so complete and also so terrifying. Then I laughed at the absurdity of a confused boy-man, sexually isolated for most of his life and celibate for half of his twenties, declaring, even prophesising his fate, his medicine, in direct action, body-based, sexual liberation.

The soured politics of healing touch; the oppressive rituals of cold hard cash; the pseudo-integrity of community, partner, solo and transcendent love; the simultaneous fetishisation and repression of erect cock; and the deliberate manufacture of gender role rigidity: these are my territories of friction and heat and priority and work. In relation to all this I am concerned about ritual containers, initiatory processes and diversity (ecological survival). I am more committed to the community than to the couple. I need help serving a greater good/god beyond ideology and morality. I want to embody and develop language for a meta-political ethic of sexual liberation.

To this gathering of remarkable homos I bring more than 10 years' training and teaching in the prayer and intentional practice of improvisational dance and performance; I bring skills of radical democracy and group process and questions about our willingness to actually live and work together; I bring the stories of thousands of men seeking wholeness and home; I bring my wounded heart, my hungry asshole, my busy brain, my ambitious cock, my salivating mouth, my scared hands, my strong and hairy thighs, my Catholic tears, my Celtic blood, my pagan cum.

Blessings to all of you for the courage and foolishness to attempt this sacred and intimate training. May my expectations and fears of you be respected. May the ancestors bless our work. May there be love amongst us. Peace.

My art and expression have so many sources. I'm an Irishman with the gift of the gab and am the fifth of six children. Because of this I want your attention now. I'm a Scorpio sun, which connects me deeply to the mysteries, especially the erotic mysteries, with a Leo rising, which calls me to express my selves in the brightest of lights.

I grew up with a strong sense of fairness and community involvement and I have experienced the collapse of political language and leftist solidarity. My performance allows me to explore issues of injustice and develop new languages, rooted in the body, to express alternative perspectives to dominant culture, violence and social control.

I have always loved dancing. In the past 20 years I have had the honour and pleasure to work with many great dancers and body-based performance artists. I sold my soul to dance. This requires a lifelong commitment to develop, reveal and teach the languages of the body. At this mid-point in my life I am sure of very little. Yet amidst this personal and social chaos I am confident that I will continue to have ideas, impulses and invitations to perform.

For many years I have complemented my performance work with research and teaching in sexual healing. Beginning in my twenties I exposed myself to the superstars of gender and sexual liberation – Joe Kramer, Annie Sprinkle, Pat/rick Califia, Betty Dodson, Fakir Musafar, Kate Bornstein. I read books, attended workshops, rituals and orgies, and spent tons of time alone thinking, touching myself, feeling and eventually learning to pray. A period of sexual initiation, a coming out as sexual, queerly sexual, and as a sexual healer, was integral to the evolution of my art. Everything changed when I allowed my sexuality to fully enter my dancing, lucid dreaming, writing and crafting of images. In my first major solo work, *Saliva* (1989), I invited the audience to spit into a hand-blown glass bowl. Receiving the bowl naked, in a cathedral-like setting under an old freeway, I added black pigment and nonoxynal-9 and then with my hand I used the communal saliva of 100 people to paint a design on my body. At the height of AIDS grief and hysteria I asked myself, and everyone, to remember when our body fluids could heal.

Central to my life and work is the integration of sexuality, activism, spirituality and creativity. I dig and dig into the context and process of my artistic choices. Noticing daydreams, paranoid or sexual fantasies, political analysis, family discussion and contemplative practice I track the interdependence of my artistic images. I notice the reverberations in my work of a global economic context, my particular class history, my shifting age and changing body, cycles of the sun and moon, whether or not I have a lover, current trends in political activism, aesthetics or advertising, and so much more.

I am a political animal. My primary sense seems to be an attention to power, equality, justice, betrayal, co-operation and consensus. After a very brief flirtation with electoral politics I chose art, specifically performance, as my primary focus and direct action. The city streets, political issues and public consciousness remain at the forefront of my creative exploits. Revel in art's potential to explore on multiple levels what activism often reduces to polarised positions, dismissal or petty fighting.

I grew up Catholic in a mining town in northern Ontario, Canada. In my family there was no talk, good or bad, about sex, intimacy or love. Gay people did not exist in any public consciousness. Though I was called a fag for the entirety of high school, I don't think most guys who tried to hurt me with this label actually thought that I would grow up to love having sex with men. To be a fag was to be cursed as weak and unimportant.

When I first met gay people, around the age of 16, I didn't identify with them. My sexual fantasies and feelings were not very specific. I was indeed attracted to girls and enjoyed kissing them. I have learned that my sexuality, like everyone else's, is unique and changing and amazing.

In general people are fearful and uninitiated in the mysteries and wisdoms of gender and sexuality. The dominant media-biased cultures delight in the confusion of girl/boy, good/bad, gay/straight dualities, which they misrepresent as a non-choice that has already been made and must be obeyed.

Sex-magic is the art of balancing and integrating duality and complexity. Sex-magic is learnt through curious play, ruthless enquiry and challenging practice. Being limited by strict roles of sexuality and gender expression does not lead to magic or healing. To heal is to make whole, is to embrace all. Discovering the inner man, woman and child is only the beginning. Try exploring and integrating the inner and outer butch, femme, monk, whore, healer, perpetrator, destroyer and exhibitionist.

Taoism, the ancient and contemporary practice from China, gives us the gift of the yin/yang, which illustrates duality in motion, each containing the other, swirling around a common centre, creating a whole. Teenagers the world over are attracted to this image. I think their psyches respond favourably to this image, which is so radically opposite to the culture of gender roles and sex oppression that squeezes youth into extremely limited spaces to express themselves and doles out harsh punishments for colouring outside the lines.

When I felt most pressured to choose a sexual identity I chose bisexual because I felt that it was the box with the most interesting and diverse people. There were more anarchists and performance artists and feminist sex workers in the bisexual box, so I felt more at home. I also thought that the bisexual box was not very clearly defined, so it seemed like the fewest people in the largest possible space.

During the bisexual revolution of the late eighties I found myself alienated from the increasing militancy of bi identity. I felt the box get smaller and more crowded. Simultaneously I was challenging my own internalised homophobia and I questioned my resistance to claiming gay and fag as an identity, especially since they more clearly represented my primary sexual practice, being a guy who enjoyed having sex with guys.

At this time the word 'queer' came to prominence, not without some ongoing controversy, and I found a new space. It was more inclusive and more widely defined. Queer was a liberating identity for me. I got to associate myself with all manner of sexual and gender diversity while simultaneously enjoying a mass political solidarity, for being queer was to be in resistance to anything that someone else thought we should be.

Mostly I think labels are as comforting as they are dangerous. Freedom is not about labels, although I think the path of liberation does involve self-definition and the intentional taking of names and joining of communities. At our best we strive to be ourselves, unique in our genius, beauty and potential, within a global network of families and communities, places where we feel at home.

As an artist I have felt the most inspired and free when I am testing the bounds of my families and communities. I think that artists have a responsibility not only to give voice to their history and community but also to expand that voice, through experimentation and integration. I am most drawn to artists who transgress genres and identities to reveal new perspectives and potential of human behaviour and expression.

My current work is all over the map. I live half the time in

France, where I tour as a performer in a French-American mongrel circus company called Cahin-Caha, *cirque bâtard*. Our show integrates circus arts with dance, performance and live music in a surreal festival of images exploring war, sex, God and their relationship to the fall. There's a lot of falling in our show. When I'm in San Francisco I live and work at 848 Community Space, which is a multi-use, easy-access, alternative culture space that hosts rehearsals, performances, dance jams, exhibits, community rituals and celebrations, erotic healing events, meetings and anything we can dream up.

In late 2000 I directed an experimental performance for a group of teenagers at the SF Museum of Modern Art. I tend to create one large-scale teen spectacle annually. My current obsession and vision is to buy a building in San Francisco or nearby to host a permanent community of artists and activists. The site would combine a low-income housing community with a circus-compatible rehearsal/performance space, a dance studio/ritual temple and additional spaces for exhibits, workshops, hot tub, garden and offices. I continue to work, both in SF and on tour, as a teacher of contact improvisation, performance creation and queer sex ritual.

EXERCISE: SOLO SEX RITUAL – JERKING OFF AS A TOOL OF PERSONAL RESEARCH AND HEALING

In my late twenties this type of dynamic, sexual meditation (Annie Sprinkle calls ritual masturbation 'Medibation' and Joe Kramer uses the term 'Soloving') became an important process of my self-discovery and directly supported my emergence as a performance artist. Several of my performance texts and images had their source in extended jerk-off rituals and the wisdom of the hard cock.

This solo sex ritual is about containing energy, expanding feelings, deepening self-awareness and combating self-censorship.

- Set aside three to five hours for this ritual.

- Buy coconut, almond or any oil you like, warmed up and coating your dick.
- You'll need a cock ring (any kind) and some 2-foot strips of fabric for binding your cock and balls. I like black cotton lycra because it's soft and stretchy. When I was younger I once used a tie of my dad's. Leather laces hold tighter than any fabric but will rip your hair out unless you shave your balls and the base of your dick.
- Over my bed I like to throw a sheet that I save for these occasions. Sculpt a beautiful sacred environment with mirrors, flowers, candles, porn art, poetry and any kind of inspired images, mementoes or objects.
- Get water and juice and some food to sustain you.
- Get something to piss in so you don't leave the room once you've started. Since we intend to be hard for the whole time, it's best to piss ahead of time, or get into the pleasure/pain of stroking a cock that wants to piss and cum but can't do either.
- Get paper and pens or pencils. Use tools you like to write or draw with.
- Take all your clothes off.
- Start consciously breathing. Deep, full breaths. If this is unfamiliar to you, just start to pay attention to your breathing. Notice how the body breathes. What expands, falls, stretches, releases. Notice the journey of the air going in and out. As you get comfortable, begin to take deeper breaths. And keep breathing. Use rhythmic music to remind you to keep breathing deeply. Try putting a sign on the wall: 'Breath'.
- Look at your naked body in the mirror. Look in your own eyes and tell yourself some version of: 'I want to be free. I want to be who I am. I want to surrender to my desires. I want to feel and I want to know what I'm feeling. I want to know my truth. I want to live my truth.' Dedicate this solo sex ritual to anything that is important to you. Sometimes I dedicate my sex play to the pleasures of future generations. If nothing comes to mind, dedicate the ceremony to discovering what is important to you. Accept the possibility of change and healing.

- Keep breathing.
- Acknowledge the universal context of your solitude with invocations. Invocations call external and internal powers to bless, protect and charge the ritual. You can invoke the elements – powers of air, fire, water, earth – or any other elemental system, with words or with the elements themselves. You can invoke your sexual mentors, ancestors or heroes with poems, quotes, pictures, or spending a moment thinking about that person or community. You can invoke Hermes, Mercury, Legba or complementary hard-on deities from any tradition: gods of the gateway, sex tricksters, messengers from the other worlds. Ask him to guard the doors of your room and soul. Offer him gifts of food, drink, sweat, spit, cum. Trade him the outcome of this ritual – your improved self in service to the world's pleasure and wisdom – for his guidance during it.
- Massage your whole body with the warm oil. Focus on relaxing, on getting involved with your body, on pleasing yourself. Invite yourself to get hard. Invite your blood to fill your cock and make it hard. Invite the phallic energy to bless you with its presence. Keep breathing and keep massaging and oiling your body until you've touched yourself everywhere. Spend extra time honouring any part of you that's tense or ugly or fat or wrong or secret. Everyone has these parts. Everyone. Your body in ritual is sacred. Healing and deep pleasure come when we honour the whole. The whole body includes all the secret parts, the heart, the spirit and soul, the desires and fears, the talents and obsessions. Keep breathing and touching and accepting.
- Now focus on your balls, perineum, anus, cock. Use lots of oil, more than makes sense. Try talking out loud, describing what you see. Squeeze your dick hard and then try very light touches. Explore with your hands and eyes. If you've been circumcised check out your scar. Circle a finger on your butthole with increasing pressure. Does it feel different while massaging the head of your dick? Explore your balls. Stretch the skin and play with

possibilities. Even though you have touched your genitals thousands of times you can learn something new right now.

- Take your strip of fabric or whatever and tie it around your cock and balls. Tie it pretty tight. Stroke your dick and watch it get more red and swollen. More full of blood. Experience the direct link between heart and dick. The body is a whole system. Find your pulse in various places – wrist, throat, thumb, ankle, asshole, chest. Fluid and electrical networks unite the body. Jerking off with deep breathing heightens the systems of the whole body. This heightened state of activity and awareness – activated by conscious practice of sex, heart, mind and soul – is the goal of this ritual.
- From here on the ritual is pretty loose, with two complementary processes to explore: (1) Keep breathing and massaging your body and stroking your dick and exploring variations of binding your cock and balls. And of course do not ejaculate for at least two hours. We are trying to build energy and channel it into creativity, insight, imagination, compassion, wisdom and healing (2) Write. Memories, sexual images, fantasies. Write lists: What do you want? What do you hate? What do you want to know more about? Who have you kissed? Who do you miss? Close your eyes and daydream. Let your own magic wand hypnotise you – what do you see? As you are stroking your body and looking in the mirror allow images and ideas that emerge to lead you to writing. Try to write while touching yourself – squeezing your dick, circling your belly, pulling your balls, stimulating anywhere and everywhere.

The key words here are play and improvisation. One image leads to another, one sensation leads to another. Do what you want. Let your mind wander. Be aware that your own mind may try to trick you into limiting what you do or think. Resist this. Continue to tell yourself that this is a non-censorship, free-sexual-expression zone. Let there be no rules to govern how you write or imagine or touch. Your writing may lead you into comments on what you're doing, childhood memories, violence, sad feelings, theories, surreal dream images, reminders to call a friend or do the dishes. Write everything down and let yourself be taken by the writing. If a new thought emerges halfway through a sentence, go with it, especially if it takes you into uncharted, unexpected images. Observe your breathing and feel your pulse (especially in your blood-trapped dick) to get cues about yourself. Write down what you physically feel in the moment. Take breaks to drink and eat and gaze in the mirror. Keep some version of the cock ring on the whole time (unless you just HAVE to pee, then do what you need and then rebind). Let the body and the mind dance. Roll into unusual shapes to see all of yourself in the mirror. Get curious about your whole self and all your beauty.

- When you're 20 or 30 minutes from stopping, put full attention into getting as high as possible. More warm oil, lots of stroking and full breathing. Take yourself into a full-body, moaning, writhing orgasm. Continue to touch, slap, rub and move your whole body as the orgasm builds. Don't rush. Stop direct dick stimulation several times and use breath and touch to get your whole body tingling. Go further and higher in your feelings. Don't ejaculate until you absolutely must. Push yourself. Breath more.
- When you are a mess of sensation and feeling, unbind yourself and cum onto your body, into your mouth or onto your page. Start writing as soon as possible after you cum. Write whatever occurs to you. With your other hand, rub your cum on your body, especially where it's never been – up your ass, in your mouth, in your hair. And write some more. What are you doing, feeling, imagining, missing, wanting? Write this.
- Stop when you wish. Thank the phallus for visiting. Thank the gods and mentors and elements for their guidance and protection. Acknowledge their tricks, that this wasn't what you expected and yet it was what you were looking for. Thank the ancestors for all their jerking off and inspiring work. Look at yourself in the mirror. Touch yourself one last time, sliding hands from head to toe, letting the ritual end and thanking yourself, your body and thanking for your body, for this luxury and rite of pleasure. Begin to release the energy and intensity of this ceremony

into your room, your house, your community, the earth, the universe. Celebrate the sensations, insights, fantasies and emotions that have come through you. Know that this power is always available to you. It is your birthright.

- Clean up with care. Eat some good food or take a bath or take a walk. Do things that shift your energy. We benefit from ongoing practice in clear beginnings and clear endings.
- You may want to do follow-up writing after a night's sleeping and dreaming. Later you can read everything. String together your favourite lines. Write an essay from the main themes that emerge. Write a coming-out letter, a response to someone with whom you need to communicate, a performance text. Follow a memory, or a fantasy, into further writing and research. Sometimes the reading and writing will get your dick hard and you can start all over again. Sometimes the reading and writing will make you sad or mad and then you'll have a good reason to start all over again...

Panos Couros

Panos Couros was born in Adelaide, South Australia in 1960. He is a screen-based sound designer, composer and arts event manager. For 17 years he has worked as a composer and sound designer, doing sound design for theatre and dance, interactive CD-ROMs, sound design and installation.

Over the past 10 years Panos has conceived, directed and produced six experimental mixed-media, multi-screen/staged, performance/installation events in Sydney, Lismore, Brisbane and Rockhampton. His audio works include the sound installations A Noise of Worms *(with Wayne Stamp) at the Museum of Contemporary Art in Sydney (1995);* Sudden *at the Institute of Modern Art in Brisbane (1996) and a rainforest soundscape along Circular Quay for the Festival of Sydney (1992).*

His past works for theatre and dance include the score for Thwack, *a solo work choreographed by Garry Stewart for the Sydney Dance*

Company (1995); #14, a collaborative multimedia event at Spring Hill Baths, Brisbane (1997); Helmet, *choreographed by Garry Stewart (1996) and* Inhabitation #2, *a dance work by Tess de Quincey (1999).*

Between 1997 and 1999 he composed sound designs for the CD-ROMs Basilisk *and* A Universe of Dirt *by Wayne Stamp and Lloyd Sharp and* Dream Kitchen *by Leon Cmielewski and Josephine Starrs, and is currently finalising the sound design for the interactive CD-ROM* Praeternatural *by Michele Barker. In late 1999 he also produced a* son et lumière *event in Rockhampton called X.*

Panos is currently employed as General Manager at dLux media arts.

My primary creative outlet is as a composer and sound designer, but not in a conventional way. I have a deep urge to express the beautiful and the ugly in the world, but mostly the beautiful. There is often a sexual aspect to my work, but this sexual motivating factor comes from the spiritual aspect of my sexuality.

I am fascinated with sound, we engage differently with it than we do with words or images. When we look at a painting, it is visual and we engage with it in a rational part of our brain. This is also true when we hear words in a spoken performance. But when we hear sound we engage emotionally with it, it is heard and responded to by a different section of our brain – with sound we are in the realm of the emotions, and that is what makes it so powerful.

There is a chakra connection with sound, and this is different for different sounds. Good music stimulates the chakras in a positive way, for example heart chakra music makes you feel beautiful. Traditional Indian music is heart chakra music, but a good, sad pop song also involves your heart. I really dislike fake music, what I call 'handbag' music, sound and songs that are mechanical and without any spirit, such as mainstream pop-dance music. Most commercial dance music made for nightclubs falls into this category. To call it 'dance music' is a misnomer because real dance music will have you tapping your fingers, moving your feet and you will find you are dancing before you even realise you are.

In 1995 I did a major three-month work with Wayne Stamp at the Museum of Contemporary Art in Sydney. We created an 8-metre-long sewerage pipe across the front lawn of the museum, right next to a real construction site, and of course everyone thought our pipe was part of the building works. Our pipe had a speaker in it, and we composed a work that was low in frequency and resonant, sounds which evoke a feeling of calm and wellbeing.

However, through this sound installation ran the sound of male-to-male fellatio. This was at the height of the 'porn on the Internet' debate, which I felt had become hysterical in tone. So while there was a huge media debate happening about how to save kiddies from being exposed to X-rated material, here was our humble pipe broadcasting explicit homosexual sexual noises every day to the lunchtime crowds at Circular Quay. All people knew was that the pipe emanated calming, soothing sounds and I think having a sexual element underlying that was a wonderfully subversive act. During the day I enjoyed watching the very hetero men straddle the pipe, sitting on it to eat their lunches, oblivious to the sounds echoing underneath them.

My current work is an interactive sound installation based on the traditional Greek story of the Oracle of Delphi, which I have called *Omphalos* (Greek for 'navel') or *Oracle No. 7*. I hope to have it installed in a Greek Orthodox Church, which will give the installation the sacred air it deserves. As you first approach *Omphalos* you will hear the sound of nine priestesses singing and see a series of traditional Greek urns arranged in a circle. Participants are encouraged to go to an urn and speak into it, asking the oracle a question. Sensors set up in the exhibition will register your approach to the urn and it will ask you what you want to know. When you ask your question, it will be echoed as a whisper from the other urns and sophisticated software will interpret your question and give you an answer.

Although I am primarily sexually attracted to other men, I regard myself as 'try-sexual' in that I will try anything as long as you don't label me over it. When I was on the board of the Sydney Gay and Lesbian Mardi Gras in 1988–89 I was primarily involved in the Mardi Gras festival and we had lots of debates about what was 'gay', what was 'lesbian' and qualified to be included in a gay and lesbian cultural celebration. One of the things I always wanted to say, but didn't, was that I wanted us to drop these labels altogether.

Labels oppress and limit us. I believe that sexuality is inherently polymorphous, that it belongs in all areas of life and can be expressed in all sorts of ways. To try and encapsulate the complex matrix that is human sexuality is as ludicrous as trying to build a bridge to the moon. For me the only use of a label for my sexuality is if someone wants to fuck me.

Here's a good sexual morality tip: don't indulge in sexual denigration. I get very annoyed when I hear sexual name-calling, such as the ubiquitous 'slut' and 'whore'. Next time you hear someone calling someone else a slut point out that it is the slut that has more courage to sexually express themselves. I believe sluts are inherently courageous people who are trying to fulfil their sexuality. Yet 'slut' is used as an insult, or to induce sexual shame, and to get the offending, highly sexual person back in their place. It uses sexuality as punishment, yet sexuality is the best healing tool. When you are sad it is certainly better to go out and have a good fuck than sit around moping.

When I was 22 I was living in a group household in Adelaide with two female sex workers. They introduced me to the reality of sex work, that it wasn't something that was 'bad' and 'corrupting' to your soul. Soon after, I went to work for a male agency in Adelaide and continued to do sex work after I moved to Sydney. It certainly was an interesting way to earn a living. I had a high libido, so having sex with multiple men a day was not a problem to me, and I thoroughly enjoyed my work.

My attitude to my clients was clear-cut – they paid for my body, but I gave them the bonus of getting my charm, spirit and personality for free. I met a lot of lonely men who wanted company and I felt for them. I think this was why I was popular, had many regular clients and was enjoyed more than many of the other boys. Ultimately, like many other sex workers, it affected my personal life because after a day 'hard at it' (so to speak) I was less sexually forthcoming with my boyfriend than I otherwise might have been. He gave me an ultimatum: 'It's me or the work', and because I loved him I resigned on the spot and haven't worked since.

3

You Sexy Thing

What makes people seek sexual favours from someone they don't know, sexual advice from a stranger and to reassign their gender?

In this chapter the insights of a professional gigolo are revealed. Who are the clients of gigolos and what do they want from them? Interestingly, far from just sex. Although the clients obviously have sexual yearnings, their emotional needs are just as important. For the successful gigolo, to be in demand means that his skills of seduction have to be practised and refined.

Professional sex experts are more than just sexual performers. Pillow talk is often more revealing than sexual exploits, with gigolos forced to be counsellor, sometimes friend, and always a confidential ear to the women and men who pay for their services.

Just as the female courtesan has a long and proud history, so does the male gigolo; it has simply been a much more hidden one. Male gigolos are usually the subject of other people's projected myths and fantasies, the ones that say they are 'getting everyone's share of sex' or living a fantasy life of all-day paid sex and mind-blowing orgasms.

Rather, many of them see themselves as professional sexual healers, performing work worthy of acclaim, not scorn. Rather than slimy characters who woo rich women, take their money and run (right on to the next woman with more money than sense), the professional gigolo sees himself as having a duty to his client.

And what about their own relationships? Their profession often compromises their need for intimacy and companionship. Many people refuse to date a male sex worker, and those who do rarely remain comfortable long term with their partner continuing to do sex work.

Good syndicated sex columnists are a rare breed, but in this chapter the 'voice of permission', as our columnist calls himself, lays bare what his letterbox reveals.

The best sex advice is practical, doesn't require years of therapy, cuts through the crap and exposes the commonality of our sexual problems. So many people write to a sex columnist only to find that their 'mortifying' sexual problem, which they could never reveal to their partner, their doctor or their therapist, is one of the top five issues preoccupying everyone.

It is important that we expand our definition of sex talk. For most men it consists of bragging or talking dirty, and not a lot of the guts of what lies in between – asking for good solid information upon which to make choices and talking honestly to their partners.

But the bottom line from our sex columnist is that you need to have courage to change, to have a new approach to your life, and to move out of your old sexual comfort zone. There is no sexual short cut to emotional growth.

Transsexualism or transgenderism, the feeling that someone has been born into the body of the 'wrong' biological gender, is a fairly new concept in the history of sexuality. It came to general public attention in the 1950s with the availability of gender reassignment surgery, primarily for male-to-female (MTF) transsexuals. Until recently MTFs had the sole public transgender profile, and indeed most people would have had no idea that female-to-male (FTM) transsexuals even existed. In the last 10 years, however, there has been an enormous coming out of FTMs, with 'tranny boys' (as they are often known) organising support groups, publications and producing some extraordinary photographic books of their gender voyage.

FTMs have fought to be recognised as part of the transgender community, despite the fact that equal numbers of men and women have always sought gender reassignment. The law in most countries has been slow to recognise transsexuals and many people have been forced to live their life in a legal nowhere land. Usually unable to alter their birth certificates, passports and social security history, many 'normal' aspects of life, such as employment, travelling abroad or marriage become a complex legal situation. Many transgender people are therefore forced to lie low, try to pass as their chosen gender and keep quiet about their sexual and gender history.

Transsexuals have been described as the 'antidote' to any overarching theories that sexual libertarians and homosexual sexual theorists might develop regarding gender. Most importantly transsexuality is proof-positive that we all experience our sex and sexuality in different ways.

Shai Shahar

Shai Shahar was born and educated in the United States, and has served in both the American and Israeli armed forces. He has lived in the Middle East and Western Europe since the early 1980s. In 1990 he moved to the Netherlands and later that year, working as a freelance journalist in Den Haag, was introduced to the owner of an escort business. He was offered a job as a gigolo and decided to take it up.

By 1995 Shai had become the most respected and successful gigolo in Holland, and was a national, if unconventional, celebrity. In July that year he co-led the controversial and highly publicised experiment in which he and three other male escorts displayed themselves in Amsterdam's famous red light windows. The aim of the experiment was to see whether women would publicly hire their 'services' if given the opportunity. The answer was a resounding 'yes'!

Since then Shai has given extensive media interviews, both nationally and internationally, and a documentary of his life has been made. He has been a frequent and popular guest on television. Although officially retired from sexual service he still devotes the majority of his time to highlighting sexual issues, is a featured columnist for a national magazine, Kim's Kontacts, *and hosts his own national radio show on Q-Radio 1224 AM/FM-cable. He is the editor, art co-ordinator/layout designer and 'techie' behind the Web site http://come.to/coracoracora.*

After being sexually active for 20 years, in which time I had travelled extensively, lived in five countries on three continents, been married, fathered a daughter and fought a war, I had resigned myself to being an 'ex-pat' in Europe. I was 35, divorced, horny and one night found myself talking to a charming redhead at a summer's evening, semi-diplomatic ball.

We went to her place afterwards and had a much less formal 'ball' of our own and then, as fate would have it, she told me of a service that was looking for 'a few good men'. She handed me a phone number for a privately run escort agency catering to discreet women of means with 'certain needs' I might be able to fill. This was not just sex, but did include sex.

I decided that I had absolutely nothing to lose. I had no moral objections to the idea, no sexual inhibitions, a natural curiosity and a sense of adventure – and importantly, only $400 in the bank with my rent due – so I dialled the number.

Many people think of gigolos as being men with a perfect life, with all their financial needs being taken care of, but there are down sides, and they can be financial, too. The easiest way to trap yourself in a sex job is to spend money as easily as you make it. I spent a lot on new clothes and a nightlife, as it is important to establish an 'identity' and a relationship with bartenders and doormen at A-list clubs, hotels, after-hours spots. They don't have to know what you do, but by the third or fourth 'date' they may guess. They don't really mind as long as you keep tipping well.

As soon as I had enough to pay my rent three times over, I moved to an apartment that cost twice as much, in a better neighbourhood, with a better view. I thought it was more 'me', whoever that was! But I did bring my daughter over to Holland to visit a few times and I was able to run a six-piece jazz band on the side. So the money I made allowed me to live the high life for a while.

Of course I was hard-pressed to explain my sudden cash flow, and people will suspect you of worse things than being a gigolo if you don't tell them. So I finally told all my friends what I was into and promptly lost half of them.

The real down side, however, was emotional. It's hard not to get emotionally tangled, or numbed, after six years of listening to so many, many terrible personal stories and having to get my dick up for women I would never have had sex with otherwise. More importantly for me I was not able to share my own emotions and stories with a partner of my own, a woman who could be my soul mate. It made me feel lonesome, despite all the beds I was sharing and the sex I was having. In the end I found I was working to maintain my new standard of living.

On a personal note, imagine if instead of 'love thine enemy', which is good advice, but has never been easy, we changed it to read 'seduce thine enemy'? See the difference? It seems to me the greatest way to stop war is to do just that, for it's hard to imagine trying to fight one with your pants down.

By studying and applying the art of seduction widely I believe we could bring peace on earth in no time. Seduction should be the highest valued skill of any diplomat. If either Albright or Milosevic had been good at it we could have been spared the nineties.

Men need to learn that women appreciate reading, writing and dancing. When it comes to magazines and books, women read more than men, just ask Oprah! They tend to be more aware of new trends and family issues than men, and are not far behind men in Internet usage for recreation or political involvement.

I do not suggest you run out now and buy the top 10 on Oprah's must-read list, but do buy – and read – a few issues of *Cosmo, People, Vogue*, and *Psychology Today* too. You will have the opportunity to get all the right answers in the quizzes you find in the other ones, and to help you understand your more 'eccentric' dates.

Part of the whole flirting game is to drop little notes into the hand, or the purse, to be read at a later moment. Again, too direct is a no-no. Notes should be suggestive but subtle. Double-entendre sentences can be left for clarification later, say, over dinner? And a variety of daring sentiments can now be found in greetings cards available in shopping malls. However, seduction includes at times the more personal touch of creative writing. With a letter you get to display your intuitive knowledge of her needs and nature or your keen observations of her more endearing features and habits.

Daring to write down one's true sexual intentions is not something we do much of any more unless we're on a chat line and talking to 'anonymous'. A letter gives you the chance to create pictures in her head that she can see over and over again and will add to her anticipation of the next meeting. Certainly it displays initiative, and gives her a sexual reflection of herself through your eyes. It need not be explicit, but hey, every woman has a fantasy, so dare to choose your words well. A thesaurus might help if you're looking to replace words like 'boobs', 'tits', 'jugs', 'cock', 'pussy', or the term 'bitch in heat'.

But in the end everything a woman needs to know before making up her mind about you will be revealed on the dance floor, be it in a disco or a bistro. Your ease, self-confidence, sensuality, virility or posturing will be obvious to her within the space of about two downbeats and a hip swing.

Because it is s-o-o-o sexually stimulating dancing was banned at times, and in many cultures certain styles of dancing still are. Think of seduction as sexual advertisement, consider dancing as the horizontal bop and consider taking lessons if you're not a 'natural' but want to appear to be. In the end you probably will.

Right now I'm attempting to make my hobby as a professional big-band jazz-swing vocalist, or a crooner, into a career. I love Cole Porter, Howard Arlen, Gershwin and my dream is to be an entertainer. An Internet-based CD-ROM music magazine, www.spinningcircle.com, has sampled a few tracks from my demo on their volume no. 3.

In the meantime I model occasionally, most recently for Accu.2 watches (I'm the guy called 'the sex machine' on the sofa in the white socks) and I have appeared in television documentaries in Holland on many subjects, even the Ten Commandments. I have had the time to explore my celebrity-induced sexual opportunities, write a book, do talk radio and learn the art of building Web sites.

Most important is that I have been able to bring my daughter to Holland for a year to bond with her, and to restore a long-lost sense of belonging to a family again, and playing daddy for real. Also I am proud to be the full-time stepfather to Aida, Cora's quite alluring daughter, who is well on her way to becoming an irresistible 'seductress' herself, someday – wait and see!

The hardest part of leaving my life as a gigolo was convincing my fellow sex workers and the media that I was really retiring, as given my reputation it took them by surprise.

TIP: How to seduce a woman

Learning how to seduce a woman is an essential life skill. Seduction is important because at the heart of seduction lies respect for the humanity, and not just the sexuality, of the object of your affection. Does that sound too politically correct? Or how about this: seduction is important because it makes every day a little bit more interesting, and the world more fun and full of opportunity. And it's safe sex!

Half of seducing a woman is merely being a gentleman, not a macho Chippendale-Johnny Bravo type. Being a gentleman means being polite, opening the door for her, standing when she enters the room or returns to the table, lighting her cigarette, if she smokes – it is the little things. Or letting her take the sexual initiative if it suits her, at least at first. It means paying attention to body language, anticipating and listening. The other half of seduction is to relax and enjoy whatever activity you happen to be sharing, like a meal, a movie, a dance, a public outing or a kiss.

Too many men jump the gun, and are either too verbally or physically direct too soon. So don't try copping a feel between courses, or unhooking her bra in the cinema, unless it's part of a game you have both agreed to play. Quite frankly, most women prefer a bit of wooing before they get to screwing, and to be a good gigolo you're going to have to understand women, or at the very least the reasons they call gigolos to begin with.

Dan Savage

Dan Savage has been writing Savage Love, *an internationally syndicated sex advice column, for nine years. The column runs in the* SF Weekly, The Village Voice, New Times Los Angeles, Chicago Reader, HK Magazine *(Hong Kong) and more than 35 other papers around the world.* Savage Love *is read by up to 4 million people each week. Dan's frank, practical approach to sexuality and relationships has sparked debate on subjects ranging from women's orgasms, safe sex and abusive boyfriends to Christians and gerbils.*

Dan is also an associate editor of The Stranger *newspaper in Seattle. He is a regular contributor to* This American Life *on national public radio and is the author of* Savage Love: Straight Answers from a Queer Sex Columnist *and* The Kid: What Happened After My Boyfriend and I Decided to Go Get Pregnant, *which recently won the PEN Award for creative non-fiction and has been optioned for TV/film.*

Dan contributes to numerous publications including the New York Times Magazine, Travel and Leisure *and* Rolling Stone *and online publications such as* Nerve.com *and* Salon. *He also appears weekly with his mother in an online Q & A on Onhealth.com. He lives in Seattle, Washington.*

In the column I write the role that I play, and that people want me to play, is a 'permission dispenser'. People write to me and say, 'I want to do this, but I worry about being normal and worry what my girlfriend or boyfriend will think, what should I do?' My response inevitably is for them to do it. If they have always wanted to do it and it's not going to go away, and if you are not hurting anyone, go ahead. I ask, 'Why are you so obsessed with being normal?'

I think by being gay I am in a good position to say that to straight people because before I could kiss anyone I wanted to kiss I had to confront and overcome huge obstacles around my sexual identity. I had to embrace the area of what is 'normal' and give myself permission to violate all sorts of taboos, before I could even leave my house and be a sexual person.

Straight people don't have to confront this area in the same way, but maybe someone is a cross-dresser or they want to get a spanking and they feel they can't come out and do this, so I encourage them not to be so concerned with what other people think. Before a gay person can even embark on the most conservative sex they have to climb this huge mountain that straight people don't have to.

There are three sexual identities to chose from: gay, straight and bisexual, and none of them is a perfect fit. There are different times in people's lives when they will identify in ways that seem truer for them than at other times in their lives. For example, a girl in her twenties might have been bisexual, but then gets married to a man and has children and 15 years have gone by and she hasn't had a same-sex experience. She might feel like she is lying if she says she is bisexual.

When you choose a sexual identity you are trying to communicate something. It is describing a desire, behaviour and choice. I feel it is important to choose a sexual identity – gay people have to label themselves so that other gay people can find them. The statistics are that gays are only 1 per cent or

2 per cent of the population. Our sexual identity is not handed to us on a platter the way straight people's sexual identity is.

There is an act of self-creation with this knowledge. Straight people often feel that gay people know more about sex and I think this is true across the board, because sex is what makes us 'not straight' so we have to think and read about it more, otherwise we don't know who we are.

I have seen tremendous changes in sexual attitudes during the nine years I have been writing my column. There is a new form of sexual openness, which came about from the Monica Lewinsky scandal, proving that Americans were actually more sophisticated than the media led us to believe. Humour is the best approach to sex, you now see things on TV that you could have only read about in my column years ago.

TIP: How to seduce a man

This is like riding a bicycle downhill, it is very easy. Any man who tells a woman they are into romantic candle-lit dinners and walks on the beach is lying. Men are aroused by danger, conflict and stress. The best way to seduce a man is to be dangerous and to seem a little threatening.

For a gay man who is trying to pick up another gay man it is very easy. Communication is the most important thing to do to improve your sex life. It is important to communicate in a way that is honest, but also sexy. Sometimes people can be clinical and cold about sex, and that can take the eroticism out of it.

For heterosexuals, once they have consented to having sex then they get down to business, while for gays and lesbians once they have consented it is just the beginning because nothing is assumed about who is going to do what to whom. It all has to be talked about, which often means gays and lesbians are good about communicating about sex.

I would encourage people to be honest about what they want with the people they are sleeping with. For example, if you are a man who requires oral sex, both giving and receiving, then you don't want to be with a woman who thinks this is a sin. By communicating early on you can part company before you have made an emotional investment in someone with whom you are not sexually compatible. It saves you getting together with someone who will make you sexually miserable.

Justin Case

Justin Case is a lawyer practising in Australia. He grew up in a happy middle-class family and has travelled the world. He was born biologically female and lived for many years as a woman. Up until a few years ago he was a dyke on a bike and heavily into SM. His quest of self-discovery and awareness took him to explore the fringes of sexuality in an effort to understand his own complex gender and sexuality.

He now lives quietly in the suburbs with his girlfriend of many years, mows the lawn on weekends and enjoys spending time with friends, his dogs and indulging in an eclectic assortment of sports and hobbies.

I don't see my gender journey as particularly extraordinary, it is just one of the things I have done in my life and part of who I am. I thought about changing my name and living as a man for many years before I actually did it. When crunch time came, and I finally made the decision that I did not want to live as a woman any longer, there were a number of factors that were at play. One of the biggest was that I just wanted to get on with my life and the constant overwhelming feeling of gender dysphoria just kept getting in the way. At times I felt as though I was always pretending to be a woman and the charade was very tiring.

I had intellectualised gender as much as I could stand; even my degree in gender theory did not help me. It did not matter how much I thought that it was OK for me to live in a gender twilight as a very butch 'woman', the bottom line was that it just felt wrong, and was increasingly difficult to maintain. Every form I had to fill in with an 'M' or 'F' option caused me such angst and confusion that it was unbearable. If I wanted to enjoy the rest of my life I needed to move on.

Having lived as a lesbian feminist one of the difficult things that I had to face was feeling like a traitor to the cause if I crossed the line and lived as a man. In the end I decided that the type of feminism I believed in did not see men as the single great evil and that there were many more complex and important issues at stake. Being born female and deciding to live as a man is probably one of the most subversive things one can do to the dominant social paradigm of strict gendered separation. Besides, it never hurt a cause to have some friends on the other side.

Having come out as a dyke I had learnt the lesson that 'those that mind don't matter and those that matter don't mind'. Coming out as being into SM was the same lesson, only deeper. Telling people that I was transgendered almost had a feeling of *déjà vu* about it. The overwhelming reaction of those who were close to me was, 'It's about time', and I have almost erased from my memory those people who freaked out.

Despite all of the love and support that were available to me from my partner, family and friends, I often felt very alone and like a freak in the world. Somehow messing with gender is sold to us as far more serious than playing around with sexuality. My self-confidence was battered and I felt very exposed. No one seemed to understand what I was going through.

My partner worked hard to help me to believe that no matter in what direction my gender went, I was a good person and worthy of her love. She also helped me see that I was being consumed by my gender dysphoria. I was becoming so swamped with the discomfort of trying to continue to live as a woman that I was literally making myself ill and losing touch with the rest of my life.

Once I made the transition and began living as a man full time I was amazed at how little I changed. Physically I changed a great deal but on the inside, emotionally and intellectually, I was the same, except that a huge weight had been lifted from me. From my first shot of testosterone I felt life coming back into me like I had not felt for many years. I was able to enjoy being me and let go of many of the things I had been supporting to protect the fragile illusion that I was coping with living as a woman. Interestingly, the first thing that slipped off was my hypermasculinity and aggressive/competitive streak.

Although I feel the same, the fact is that the world treats me very differently now that I am seen as a man. As I learn to function in society as a man the everyday differences between how men and women are treated, and the forces that shape male behaviour, are frighteningly clear to me.

While I was living as a woman I played, for a time, in the deep end of the SM community. There I found men, women and trannies who determined their view of me as a sexual creature based on the type of kinks we had in common rather than what sex I was born. This is very different to the usual model of first judging what sex someone is and then deciding if they are straight or gay. At the boundaries of sexuality gender is very blurry and not all that important, because on a scale of kinkiness gender fluidity is fairly low. I was able to dress, act and fuck like a man (however that is) and no one in that community saw this as particularly odd.

SM sexuality demands a high level of self-awareness. You really need to think about what you are doing and consciously ask yourself why you are doing it. The need to openly talk about taboo issues, such as sexual desire, in order to work out consent gives you language and tools to think about other difficult issues, including gender. Talking openly to people about very personal things, sometimes people I hardly knew, required me to really think about who I was and what I wanted.

Sexuality and gender are different things but they are linked in many ways. I think that in exploring the extremes of sexuality I was, at least in part, searching for a space that embraced my gender fluidity and for the language to describe it. As a part of the SM community, particularly in San Francisco, I was able to express my masculine gender and express a form of sexuality that transcended gender. For me this was a very important part of coming to terms with my need to live as a man. It was also a time of very hot sex.

I am in a committed relationship that began well before I began living as a man. Our deep love and the fact that we are compatible as people has not changed; just about everything else probably has. Sexually we have both changed. I think that this is a product of both my gender transition and independent changes in my partner's life. We have both grown a great deal in this relationship and one of the ways I have grown is through my gender change, but this does not diminish the other changes we have both been through.

The issues that partners of transgender people face are often overlooked. Much of the literature on partners focuses on how they can support someone going through a transition. As my partner pointed out, this is all very well but fails to address the issues she was being forced to face herself for no reason other than that she was my partner. Transgendered people bring to a relationship a whole bucket of sticky gender issues that a non-transgendered person would otherwise not have had to deal with.

When we met, my partner had just come out as a lesbian, and her relationship with me was a lesbian relationship. She had also declared that she was over having relationships with men. So my decision to live as a man made this a bit tricky for her, to say the least. She had to do a lot of thinking about her queer identity and how this fitted in with my new masculinity. She had to deal with people saying that she was not a 'real' lesbian, as well as people saying she could not get a 'real' man. In the same way that I had to deal with the feeling that people would think I was Mr Freak, she had to cope with being Mrs Freak.

One of the things that caused tension was me wanting to choose who I told about my transgendered status. She felt she needed to tell people as a way of maintaining her queer identity, because the world was increasingly seeing her as straight. I believe that the way we stayed together through my transition and beyond was through a deep trust in our love and constant work on our communication skills. I think that, in the end, the period of my transition has brought us closer together. With the skills honed at that time we have faced other challenges together and I hope that we will continue to do so evermore.

My relationships with men have changed a great deal. When I was living as a butch leather dyke most men appeared, frankly, afraid of me. I don't mean that they were physically afraid of me, but more that they were intimidated by what I represented. I guess that many straight men see butch leather dykes as being all that they are, but more, and as having access to a sexual world that they don't (except in fantasy). Butch dykes are perceived as having access to femme women and leather dykes as having access to the world of BD/SM women that most men are only shown in pornography.

To many, the image of a butch leather dyke is of a powerful creature, beyond men's reach and enjoying a world that revolves around sex and does not involve any boring stuff like family responsibility. The men that I was friends with in that period of my life were almost all gay leather men and I was close enough to them so that they knew my life was not really all that different to anyone else's. I still had stresses and worries, and not everything in my world was about sex. Although of course we all knew that I was having better sex than any of them!

When I was in the period of transition I think that men were also threatened by me. After all, if a woman could become a man what was left that was special about men? Now I am just one of the blokes. Most people have no idea that I used to live as a woman. I don't present a threat to anyone's masculinity any more. I know lots of men and would count a few as friends. I still find it difficult relating to other men in some situations. I think my female upbringing, and my first-hand experience of how systemic discrimination operates, give me an insight into the world that most men will never share.

Physically I am stronger and healthier than I have ever been. The surgeries I had were a bit of a drag, but I have no regrets. Psychologically I think I am a whole lot calmer, more 'centred', to be New Age about it. Living as a woman I always had something to prove. I was hypermasculine. Without realising it at the time I was very competitive and aggressive. I had to be the leader of the pack, literally and figuratively (I was head of the local chapter of dykes on bikes and had the biggest, meanest Harley one could have). Now I have nothing to prove. I am very relaxed in my masculinity and far more comfortable with my feminine side than ever before. In fact, I am so non-competitive and non-aggressive that the question that most people have of me is, 'Are you gay?' By the way, I think this is a reflection on sexual and gender stereotypes, not on gay men.

One thing that has not changed is my personal values and these are deeply affected by having been raised female. I have a consciousness of feminism and the issues that face women that those raised as male will never have. I understand women's issues and am now also coming to understand the oppressive forces on men and the cycle with which these feed back into the oppression of women. Trannies are in the unique position of being able to sit on both sides of the fence as well as the middle. Unfortunately when I talk with women about gendered oppression I am dismissed as 'just a SNAG' [sensitive

New Age guy]. If I out myself as a tranny I am equally dismissed as a traitor to the feminist cause.

While I was transitioning I was constantly surprised at how supportive and unshocked other people were. With my work colleagues and acquaintances I took the approach that they needed to know that I was making this transition and that I wanted them to refer to me using the male pronoun and my new name from now on. I told people face-to-face where I could. Almost without exception people accepted that this was how it is and after some initial curiosity and gossip everyone just got on with their jobs. I was quite amazed. I work in a fairly conservative profession and I had anticipated having to change jobs.

I maintained my involvement with the hobby and community groups that I am involved in and despite a few early pronoun slips there has been very little reaction, or at least little reaction that I am aware of. In some ways I think people are more comfortable having me around as a boy than as an obviously butch dyke. The only group from which I was rejected was the local lesbian community, but they already disliked me because of my open involvement in the SM lifestyle.

The most amazing story is probably my parents. I am extremely lucky and humbled by the depth of their love. If a group of trannies sat around and designed the most supportive parents possible, they would come up with parents exactly like mine. My parents have taken the attitude that they love me no matter what and that if this is what I need to do then so be it. They are more interested in how happy my relationship is and whether I am enjoying my job than what gender I am.

I have two tips for tranny boys. The first is to do your research. I did a lot of research about other tranny boys' experiences. I read books, searched the Internet and, where possible, talked to people. Finding out about other boys' stories helped me have an idea of what to expect and to learn from other people's successes and mistakes in their journeys. It also helped me to be mentally prepared for the journey ahead.

I also found out everything I could about how medicine and the law viewed trannies. You need to understand the medical model and to be able to explain yourself to doctors and psychiatrists in terms they will understand. Although I think that the traditional medical model of transsexuality is way off the mark, the medical profession are the gatekeepers to the drugs and surgery I wanted, so I learnt to talk their talk. I also researched the law to understand my rights and to make sure I could get my 'legal sex' changed where I could and all my documents updated.

My second tip is to remember that gender changing is not the centre of everybody's universe. Changing gender entails a massive personal upheaval in one's life and involves huge amounts of mental, emotional and physical stress. It is easy to get caught up in it and to think that the whole world cares about it as much as you do. However, as far as most of the rest of the world is concerned it is just something about you (whether they approve or not), it is not something they devote a huge amount of time to thinking about – unless of course they are your parents, children or partner. I think you need to be very patient with other people and let them come to terms with it in their own way. I have found that by just getting on with my life and being who I am other people get on with theirs and everything goes fairly smoothly. I think that if I had demanded that other people make a fuss of my gender change everything would have been a lot more difficult.

My sexual desires have become much simpler. As a leather dyke I had a very complex sexuality. I was very into exploring the boundaries, playing with dominance and submission, fantasy, pain and fetishes. I was attracted to women who shared this desire to push the limits. Since I have been taking testosterone my desires have become very simple. I just want to fuck. The other stuff would still be OK, as a diversion, but the bottom line is a lust that focuses on plain old-fashioned fucking. I look at my girlfriend with what she calls my 'goofy expression', and it means that all I can think about is rutting. It is something I find deeply satisfying. There may well be something hormone-driven about it, I don't know. I just know that for me I now feel driven to do the things that I once would have dismissed as boring.

EXERCISE: INCORPORATING A BIT OF GENDER PLAY INTO YOUR LOVE MAKING

For those that live as women I would strongly recommend grabbing a strap-on and fucking someone. Feel the power of penetrating someone and the responsibility of being on top.

For those that live as men, if you are brave enough, hand over control and responsibility to your partner. Use your imagination and role-play. Switching roles for an evening can be profound and hot.

4

Sexy is the World

Whether you like your sexual material lukewarm, soft and erotic, or totally hardcore, the adult industry that produces it has always been controversial. The sex industry has always been seen as a boys-only school, and women are just starting to make inroads into this last arena of male sexual power.

The feminist anti-pornography movement has seen the adult industry as inherently corrupt, whose agenda is to make as much money as it can, as fast as possible, with no care for the misery it inflicts in the meantime. This man's, man's, man's world is seen as the source of female oppression.

The feminist anti-censorship movement takes the opposite stand, arguing that sexism in pornography only reflects the sexism in society. They believe that women have as much right to sexual material as men, and that women need to storm this bastion of male control.

The proliferation of women's sex shops, services and products seems to indicate who is winning this feminist war of hearts and minds, but leaves unanswered a number of interesting questions. Who are the men who work in the adult industry? How do you get to be a porn star, a sex writer or a sex industry lobbyist? And are you forever corrupted by the experience?

Traditionally men who work in the sex industry have attracted very different opinions from men and women outside it. Men often assume that the men in the sex industry have a work environment where sex is on tap, the women are free and easy, and their days are spent in an orgy of sleaze.

Women are often highly suspicious of sex industry employees, assuming that they are the lowest of the low, sleaze bags who profit off the backs (literally) of women.

The men in this chapter reveal the human face behind the sex industry. Although women have written numerous books about their adventures, horror stories or comic journeys through the adult industry, rarely has the voice of men in the industry been heard.

It might surprise many to know that male porn stars have the same insecurities as other men, and work daily with almost unreasonable pressures to 'perform' on cue. Their bodies are under a scrutiny second only to supermodels, with every imperfection noted. And unlike their female counterparts they are unable to fake orgasm and ejaculation. In this case the camera truly doesn't lie!

The gay male porn industry is a significant force within the adult industry, with its own stars, video lines and erotic awards. Like women's involvement in the industry, the involvement of gay men in the manufacture of products, services and videos has lifted the standard of what is on offer.

But are the issues for gay male sex workers the same as for their straight, or bisexual, counterparts? It seems so. Genital size is the key to a brilliant career, no matter what you look like. Gay male porn seems to be divided into 1) the standard sleaze bag and 2) thinking gay man's porn, the latter epitomised by the new films of gay male porn king Chi Chi La Rue.

Interestingly, and unlike many women's perceptions, working in the sex industry has not hardened the men in this chapter's view of women. They remain touchingly loving towards the women in their lives, and if they are critical at all it is of the industry, not the women in it. Many are concerned about the treatment of women in the sex industry, and strongly support the new female forays into the adult world, as owners and operators of sex venues, sex shops and X-rated video companies. They believe that it can only make the sex industry more representative of the full spectrum of human sexuality.

The men interviewed here have worked in the adult industry over many decades. They show the mundane reality behind sex work, the often comic side to trading in sex, and what adult industry men are looking for in a relationship. Many of the sex industry men are surprisingly New Age, professing a deep belief in spiritual sex, creative celibacy and the desire to bond deeply on a soul level with another person.

Richard Pacheco

Richard Pacheco was born Howie Gordon in 1948 to an orthodox Jewish family in Pittsburgh, Pennsylvania. After university graduation, he worked in Washington, DC on programmes to help address poverty in the US. While researching the San Francisco Bay area, he visited a commune in Berkeley, California and was so taken with the lifestyle that he decided to quit his job and move in. Shortly after this time he met his wife and he has been married to her for over 25 years.

He explored his interest in acting and filmmaking at university in Ohio and began his career as a porn star in 1975. Over the next 10 years he appeared in over 100 X-rated movies and had sex on film and video with about 150 women and one Japanese vibrating mechanical fish. He won three Best Actor awards, five Best Supporting Actor Awards, was Playgirl *magazine's Man of the Year in 1979 and was chosen as Best Director by the* Adult Video News *for his 1983 film* Careful, He May Be Watching.

With the advent of heterosexual AIDS headlines in 1984, Pacheco began withdrawing from the adult film business and concentrated on a second career as a writer. Since then he has had an active role in bringing up his three children and writing for various sex journals, including Playboy Online, Libido *and* Spectator. *At present he is writing his memoirs of his years in the business, called* Hindsight.

It all started in Berkeley when my wife introduced me to sex therapy. She was training as a surrogate in Masters and Johnson's sex therapy and I would grit my teeth and say, 'Have a nice day at work, dear!' as she would go off to be with some guy. But she would come home with stories of men who were years older than us and who had never even been able to be inside a woman. After they had completed a successful round of therapy these patients were finally able to enjoy sex. Despite the difficulty and oddity of sharing my wife, I felt significant work was being done.

It was three or four years later that I started my own involvement in the sex business, but the focus was on entertainment, not therapy. Oddly enough, I had never had any sexual dysfunction occur in my private life, but when I started in the porn business, I seemed to have it all. I used to come home and talk about it with my wife, who would then coach me on how to function under pressure.

Because I went through so much sexual repression early in life, I got to the point as a young adult where I virtually exploded into sexual freedom. Looking back, I felt this was necessary just to get normal. America in the 1950s was a very sexually repressed place. I also grew up as a fat kid with the largest breasts in the seventh grade, so there was gender confusion as well as the usual traumas of puberty. I endured great amounts of teasing and tormenting from my peers. So the notion of becoming a sex star later in life, and becoming a body beautiful, was like winning an Oscar. It was a reward for the thousands of miles I ran and the hundreds of sit-ups that I did. Socially, I went from being Quasimodo to Robert Redford.

It was being touched which I believe finally made me lose weight. I had a mother and four males who hovered around her: my brother, a mentally retarded uncle, my father and myself. She was not a touch person; love came from food and I think I was overfed and touch deprived. When I finally had a girlfriend and got into preliminary sexuality, the extra weight just seemed to fall off.

From 1975 to 1985 I was a porn star and for three to four years after that I was involved in the business in a non-sexual way. My relationship with sex, and my wife's attitude, changed. In the beginning my wife thought it was something cute her husband did. By 1984 she felt it was something cute her husband had done and wished he were done doing it.

There were other factors as well. When we started a family, the outbreak of genital herpes in the late 1970s led me to decide to not work with anyone who was infected with the disease, because during a birth it could possibly lead to brain damage in a newborn.

At that time the industry was a very small community; only about 300 or 400 people made all the porn movies in America. AIDS came along and that issue finally caused me to retire. In 1984 came the first news headline of the heterosexual transmission of AIDS. It was a big decision to quit – I had come from a $25-a-day actor to a $1,000-a-day actor, and was now at the top of my career. My wife said to me, 'Don't you think one of us should stay alive to raise our children?' and that was it. I could not see my way clear of that. The way I participated in the industry was as a kid out of the sixties with a sexual consciousness of liberation and revolution. Then we all had a common sense of edginess.

The pill had really created a sexual revolution and we had easy cures for syphilis and gonorrhoea, which had been the equivalent of AIDS. That window of sexual revolution changed sexual values, but when AIDS came along, the party was over. I never thought in my lifetime I would see the sexuality flower close again, but it did, and then common sense dictated to be careful, which I was. There was a year, or year-and-a-half, before people started talking about safe sex.

In the industry itself, unfortunately, well, let's just say that it is not generally filled with the leading lights of the community. The producers and directors did not want to talk or hear about AIDS, they just wanted to pretend that it didn't exist and they weren't going out of their way very far to look after the welfare of the performers.

In 1985 and 1986 I decided to take some jobs with the few

producers who were willing to do safe sex. In the end, their sense of business was that movies with condoms did not make as much money as the ones without. During this time I was not thrilled with the idea that on the other side of this rubber [condom] is potential death.

I had always had trouble functioning sexually in front of other people, and now after insisting that the videos show safe sex, when I put on a condom, that was it. I was the one who insisted that the industry use safe sex, but when I put on the condom, my dick took the car keys and went home. If Viagra had been around when I did those sex scenes, I would have used it.

The industry is basically a young person's game. A remarkable exception to that is Dave Cummings, who is 55 or 60 years old, a former military officer and a West Point professor, who five years ago got into pornography. He now plays all the father roles.

When I was in the industry six months was a generation. A lot of women would last that long and then they would be done. Very few of the guys had a career. Men generally thought it was an easy assignment but it wasn't, and when they found a man who could do it and be reasonably successful as an actor, staying sober and turning up regularly he would get lots of work. The industry has an unquenchable thirst for new 18-year-old girls.

In the late 1970s there was a major shift in the porn industry as they started to value acting. With films like *Nothing To Hide, The Dancers, Irresistible, Sex World*, the industry was trying to compete with Hollywood, only adding full-bodied sex scenes. This blew up in the early 1980s with the video revolution. It used to cost anywhere from $75,000 to $125,000 to make a bad film, including some of the ones I was in. Oh, there were some good scenes. But I don't think a really good whole film has been made yet.

For a video today, they would spend between $2,000 and $10,000 for the same movie. When only the professionals were making the movies, they became boring because the people involved were no longer engaged in what they were doing. They were just getting through the sex scenes and were bored.

Then came a wave of amateur pornography, which was very exciting because the performers were having fun with the sex.

It took me 10 years to make 100 movies, which sounds like a lot, but I was very selective about my work. Today an actor will make 300 video movies in one year. There are so many movies being made that you can get a movie of any particular fetish you want. There are whole movies of peeing, spanking or anything else you want.

Everyone assumed that because I was a porn star I had a big penis, but I didn't. In the days of film, when the screen was 20 feet high, it wouldn't matter what size your penis was.

I have written a few scripts for porn movies and worked as an assistant director, but I found that I didn't like being on the set any more. If you are on the set of a sex film and you are not having sex you get aroused at 9 am, you get a hard-on all day and eventually you just get a stomachache.

TIP: A porn star's secrets

How to be a good lover is to ask her what she wants. Make it easy for her to talk to you and try to deliver what you honestly can, and if you start to resent it, stop. Keep the communication going. The secret to being a good lover is to follow directions. You can't communicate too much. Not everyone is right for one another. I found in the industry if I was put with a taller woman I turned into her little brother and it disengaged my erotic feelings completely. I learnt through trial and error, by being honest with myself, what my desires are. What gets you hot in your twenties may not be what it is in your thirties. A lot of people have secret desires that they don't want to admit to themselves because they are embarrassed, or it doesn't fit their politics. True eroticism has nothing to do with all that, it's not necessarily rational.

Jack Heidenry

Born and brought up in St Louis, Missouri, Jack Heidenry attended St Louis University, where he majored in theology. After a brief career as a newspaper reporter, he became managing editor of Herder & Herder in New York, the leading publisher of scholarly Roman Catholic theology and philosophy books in the US. Meanwhile he married, and had four children in six years.

In 1973 he and his family decided to drop out of society, moving first to a farm in Missouri, then to a small town in the south of England, Spain and finally to Mexico. During this period he taught his children at home, using spelling and maths textbooks bought at Woolworths, and relying on food stamps to get by. At the end of seven years of bare-bones poverty, but having enjoyed the unparalleled luxury of being a full-time dad to his children, he decided to return to the US and work as a freelance writer and editor of a new St Louis magazine.

In 1982 he moved to New York and became executive editor and eventually editor-in-chief of Penthouse Forum, *which coincided with the beginning of his professional interest in sex. He also started up a new Penthouse publication,* Hot Talk, *published a paperback,* Test Your Sex IQ *(Warner Books) and edited several collections of Penthouse erotica and letters.*

In 1989 he left Penthouse and wrote a book, Their's Was the Kingdom: Lila and DeWitt Wallace and the Story of the Reader's Digest, *published in 1993. Four years later he published* What Wild Ecstasy: The Rise and Fall of the Sexual Revolution. *He is currently editorial director of the forthcoming Museum of Sex in New York, and editor of www.theposition.com.*

I got into the area of sex, professionally speaking, quite accidentally. Back in 1982 my wife and I wanted to return to New York, where we had first lived, got married and had four children. After that period of about 10 years, we dropped out of society for most of the seventies and travelled and taught our four children at home, though not with any real seriousness. My oldest daughter didn't learn to read until she was eight, though she later attended Columbia University.

Anyway, at some point we realised it was time to return to the real world. I got a job working as an editor in St Louis, and in 1982 decided I'd become a freelancer in NYC, where my family and I still live. However, a friend heard of my plans and invited me to become executive editor of *Penthouse Forum*, the digest-sized sex information magazine published by Penthouse. He phoned and offered me the job, and I accepted without ever having even seen a copy of the magazine. Then I went out and bought a copy of the magazine. I nearly fainted. A little smut magazine, I thought. But, after all, it was a job, and I was in no position to negotiate or look elsewhere as the move was about a week away.

Up till this point, I was like many men. I assumed I knew all there was to know about sex if for no other reason than I knew how to do it, more or less. If I ever came across articles about sex, I never read them. Not that I was a prude. But I just assumed information about sex was either meant to arouse, or else was of so banal a nature as not to be interesting.

My eight years at *Forum* were a serious eye-opener, and stimulating beyond belief. I came into contact with sex professors, call girls, transvestites, pornographers and just about everyone else on the sexual spectrum. I realised that when it came to sex, I was a dummy. I knew nothing, really; I was just another dopey male. I also came quickly to understand that women knew far more about sex than men. I think this is primarily through female intuition, and perhaps also as a result of their biology; and also because they understand sex in a way men do not. For a man, getting laid is in most cases the most important thing. But for women, it is a much more complicated, richer experience, even if it's only a brief affair.

Beyond that, I realised that sexual problems are at the root of just about every evil society has. At least this is my opinion. Not just rape, battery, serial murder, but financial greed, racism and hate all have, I think, a sexual explanation at bottom. I also realised that very few people, as I once was, have any interest in sex as an intellectual discipline. Sex has been relegated to sex advice columns and wacky sex experts, or else to imponderable sexuality studies that nobody can either decipher or maintain a genuine interest in.

So when I left *Forum*, I decided to write a book about the enormous changes that have taken place in sexuality since 1965, a date more or less when numerous forces coalesced into the sexual Big Bang that came to be known as the Sexual Revolution. I interviewed hundreds of people, did the usual archival research and the result was *What Wild Ecstasy: The Rise and Fall of the Sexual Revolution*. My original title was *Sex Among the Ruins*, which I still prefer, but the publisher thought that title too negative.

The book explores four main areas: sexual research, beginning with Masters and Johnson's affirmation of the clitoral orgasm and refutation of Freud's vaginal orgasm; court cases that enlarged the interpretation of the US's First Amendment, permitting importation or publication of so-called pornography; gay and transvestite/transsexual liberation; and, fourth, the enormous sea change in popular culture as it experienced the sexual revolution.

Interestingly, my sexual studies and work hardly affect my personal relationship with my wife and children. Despite my ignorance at an intellectual level, I was always pretty liberal and non-uptight in my personal life. My children were told the facts of life when they were quite young; we never laid a Catholic guilt trip on them (my wife and I were raised Catholic); and in fact three of my four children eventually worked at *Penthouse* as editorial assistants while going to college. Bob Guccione helped to pay, you might say, for their tuition. All three loved the experience.

I was the founding editor of *Hot Talk*, which ultimately became a competitor of *Hustler* magazine. I don't know if men interested in anal sex worry about being gay; what I do know is that *Forum* received hundreds of letters every month. Unlike most magazines all of them were authentic, and we edited them only for grammar. The only letters I refused to publish regarded incest, which I regard as immoral as well as illegal. Nor did we publish the occasional letter about paedophilia or bestiality.

Most letters, by far the majority, were probably just fantasies and not strict recounts of what actually happened. Most men should be so fortunate as to experience the wild sex encounters these letters contained. I looked upon them as a form of entertainment and probably masturbatory fantasy tools. The main fantasy men talked about in their letters was watching their wife have sex with another man. Usually they are involved too, and it is a threesome. Undoubtedly these letters were in fact disguised fantasies about latent homosexuality.

However, many letters did contain outright segments about a man meeting another man, and deciding to explore a homosexual experience. I am a believer in Kinsey's estimate that about 10 per cent of the male population in the US is gay; and I went to considerable lengths in *What Wild Ecstasy* to refute a later study that tried to ascertain that the figure was actually 4 per cent.

Swinging is definitely making a comeback in the US, as in Australia. The Lifestyles Organization is booming as never before, according to founder Bob McGinley, but I guess the real sexual surprise which is happening is the coming out of transsexuals. This is happening on several fronts. The work of pioneers like Dr John Money has been challenged by many transsexuals like the Hermaphrodites with Attitude group, who think that hermaphroditism is perfectly natural, and that the sexes shouldn't be divided into the old male/female. Whether this is wise or not is another question.

There are a number of disturbing trends in the area of sexuality: a return to unprotected sex among gay men; a probable porn witch hunt under the Bush administration, with Ashcroft as attorney general. Porn do's and don'ts have already been drawn up by pornographers in anticipation of this witch hunt, eg no male-on-male anal sex.

There is growing acceptance of sexual diversity and semi-nudity in the media, and I think that the US population in general is beginning to accept homosexuals much more, but despite this the US remains a profoundly puritanical society, with no end in sight. The proofs of this are: lack of sex education in our schools, the huge anti-abortion movement, the abstinence-only campaign in our schools, the don't ask/don't tell policy in the military, *ad nauseam*.

If sex is between adults and is fully consensual, neither the sex advice business, nor the churches, nor society has any business butting in and telling them how to live their own lives or telling them how to be sexual. It often takes a lifetime for a person to understand and come to terms with his or her sexuality. The main thing we can provide is information. Information about sex practices, why most are not unusual and certainly not condemnable; information and encouragement for people to explore their sexual selves to the fullest.

Well, I don't know what the Internet has really accomplished, sexwise, except for the creation of chat rooms. 99.9 per cent of all sex sites are owned by hardcore pornographers and you have to pay for it, just as you would for a video.

There are virtually no intelligent sex sites in the US that are widely accessible and free, that I'm aware of: Nerve.com for literary erotica; Salon.com's sex channel for a pretty wide range of sex information and stories; theposition.com, rather like

Salon.com in that regard; and Cleansheets.com. That's about it, and you add up all the total viewers and you still have only a fraction of browsers. Most people on the Net still go to places like iVillage and Oxygen for sex advice and information. I can't think of two dumber sites.

I am currently working on a book on male sexual aggression and sexual violence. As I said above, sex, specifically sexual violence, is the root of all evil. What causes this violence, and what can be done to prevent it, is the subject of my book (which is still years away from completion). Putting sex criminals in jail obviously isn't the answer. We need prevention, not punishment.

Robbie Swan

Robbie Swan was born in Sydney in 1951 and has lived most of his life in Canberra. During his last year of high school he undertook classes in bible studies because he wanted to study theology at university. He decided instead to study journalism but dropped out as a draft-dodger in the final days of the Vietnam war.

He developed an interest in meditation early in his life and left Australia in the early seventies to study under the Beatles' spiritual mentor, the Maharishi Mahesh Yogi. He ended up as the Maharishi's florist and spent several years in the Swiss Alps with him.

In the mid 1970s he returned to Australia, teaching meditation and yoga. During this time he started writing freelance articles about sex, politics and spirituality.

In 1983 he was asked to edit an Australian New Age magazine called Simply Living. *In 1985 he set up his own political humour and satire magazine,* Matilda, *which became a cause célèbre in the fight against defamation laws being used as censorship tools.* Matilda*'s flame burnt strongly but quickly and the magazine went down under a welter of writs from high-profile politicians, judges, doctors and celebrities.*

He then worked in TV and radio as a producer and researcher.

In 1988 he was contracted by Australia's X-rated video industry to set up and run a political lobbying campaign against the Reverend Fred Nile's push to ban adult videos. In 1992 he met another sex industry lobbyist, Fiona Patten, and together they formed the Eros Foundation, Australia's lobby group for the sex industry, as well as a strong personal relationship.

Dressed as a woman for public appearances, he also edited a new couples' magazine called Ecstasy *and continued this hoax to promote the magazine over a six-month period. As a lobbyist and then publisher for the Eros Foundation for the last few years, he has recently taken over the running of the* Eros Journal *full time and plans to turn sex industry and censorship issues into a national interest magazine.*

He has two children from a previous marriage and lists his hobbies as gardening, music and exercise.

My involvement with Transcendental Meditation and yoga for 15 years had a lot to do with my sexual development. I was the official florist to the Maharishi Mahesh Yogi in Switzerland and became a meditation teacher in 1974. During that time I worked alongside people like John Gray (author of *Men are from Mars, Women are from Venus*) who were starting to look at modern sexuality through tantric models. At the same time there were an equal number of people in that setting who were experimenting with celibacy for a number of different reasons. It was very instructive. Although there were a few 'natural' celibates who tended not to talk much about it, the majority were 'mood-makers' who opted for a sexless life out of tension and stress. These people tended to trumpet their lifestyle loudly and wear it like a badge of honour. The 'tantrics', on the other hand, tended to hide their ideas and develop them within closed circles.

Although the intellectual understandings of Vedic spirituality and the experiences in meditation were outstanding, I filed these concepts of repression and sexuality versus celibacy away for future 'study'.

I feel that my spirituality has been a contributing factor to my sex life because when you are into meditation, your sex life develops naturally. Assuming that you are a natural 'householder' and not a natural 'recluse' or celibate, raising your spiritual life boosts your sexuality in the same way that it boosts your fitness, your intellect and your emotional life.

Without a spiritual component to life, most people tend to lose interest in sex as they get older and when female and male menopause hits at around 50, many people give it up altogether. Genuine spiritual development that delivers real transcendence may not alter the physical changes that take place in the body but it brings new horizons to one's sex life. In men, for example, although ageing brings slower and less impressive erections, orgasms can broaden out and lengthen into five- and 10-minute mind-blowing affairs. Scientific research into these areas has not even scratched the surface yet.

I believe that there are very few monks and nuns in the Christian tradition who are genuine celibates, who can live away from society and develop their spirituality in isolation from sexuality. For most of us, when we get into meditation or a spiritual lifestyle we get into sexuality as well, which is a problem for most institutions because they want to deny it. Hence the epidemic of child sexual assault in Christian institutions around the world at the moment. From the Christian churches to the Eastern religions, most of them are developing people's sexual natures, and then repressing them. It's dangerous stuff.

In 1988, while working as a journalist, I was introduced to the political arena of sexuality by Professor Paul Wilson, the then Deputy Director of the Institute of Criminology in Canberra. At that time, a very Catholic Attorney General, Lionel Bowen, was doing the Catholic bishops' bidding on morality and was going to ban X-rated videos. Paul Wilson could see that if this happened all the proceeds from the legal X-video industry (approximately A$25 million per year) would go straight to the Chinese triad syndicates, who wanted to get a toe-hold in Australia. Paul approached me to start a campaign to stop the bans. What started as a six-month consultancy then turned into a lifetime's work.

My children have been affected by the work that I have done for the sex industry. For example, I was asked to leave the school board before my time was up because I dared to dress in women's clothing. The issue had been compounding for a while with some of the local mothers, who thought that having a sex industry lobbyist on the school board was not appropriate. When I launched a new couples' sex magazine called *Ecstasy* I couldn't find a woman to edit it and so I dressed up as a mature woman editor to sell the issue. I was eventually exposed in the *Weekend Australian* magazine and clearly many people thought it was too much.

Although my children had to put up with some unforgivable comments from other children and parents about their father being a 'pornographer', I hope I taught them to stand their ground in the face of mindless political correctness. I don't work for an arms manufacturer or a cigarette or alcohol company, so I have a perfectly clear conscience. I work for an organisation that hopefully puts people in a better place in their lives and gives them more pleasure and less repression. But anyone who works for, or in, the sex industry and has children, knows that their kids suffer from malicious and bigoted slander in the schoolyard and in other community arenas.

I am lucky that my parents and the rest of my family are very sexually liberated and do not suffer from guilt or shame at all. Without this support I probably would never have gone down the road I did.

My relationship with Fiona, my partner, was pretty regular at the beginning. We fell in love and bought a house. But the difference for us is that by starting up the Eros Foundation we have worked in the sex industry together. Being around such diversity of sexuality has really opened up our own lives because on a daily basis we were forced to look at the different ways people have sex, and the sort of sexual services and products they buy.

After seven years of living and working together we felt we needed space in our relationship. I think that there are only about 10 per cent of the population that mate for life and that about 80 to 90 per cent of the population are not naturally monogamous. We had a threesome and out of this we gave each other the space we needed to explore our sexuality with others, as long as we were perfectly honest about everything.

At times it was difficult for us but we felt it was important to explore sex. What we learnt out of it was that if we felt attracted to someone else to tell each other straight away. We also used different sexual products, and became more broad-minded, rather than let our relationship run the course of jealousy and rejection.

The Eros Foundation has had an effect on the sex industry, which is Australia's newest industry. The biggest change over the past year or two has been the Internet, with two major public companies who sell sex products being listed on the Stock Exchange. They are therefore owned by the mums and dads of Australia, as John Howard [Australia's prime minister] would put it. The Eros Foundation now gets a lot of publicity, with media and politicians referring to it almost every day. The motivation for everything Eros does is to improve the quality of life for those involved in and around the adult industry.

I don't feel general sex legislation affects us, but any online legislation could. On a visit to the UK recently, Fiona and I went to the Home Secretary's office – it was the first time they had accepted a delegation from the sex industry. X-rated videos had been illegal in Britain since Margaret Thatcher's era. We spent three hours with members of the Home Secretary's advisers, vice squad and the chief film censor and lobbied them on behalf of the sex industry.

In the UK there has now been a change in the legislation covering adult products [sexually explicit adult videos became legal in 2000] and we hope we were part of the catalyst for this rethink.

In the last couple of years we have seen phone sex banned, which had been a huge industry. Many large, 'respectable' companies make money out of the sex industry without acknowledging that they do so. Since the ban, the same money is still being made, but instead of Australian companies reaping the profits, they are now being made offshore. Erotic phone lines still operate, but Howard's government has made Australia's main phone company employ actors to get on the lines to check that the conversation does not stray to sexual matters. It's very scary, this Big Brother style of legislating sexual free speech.

The sorts of sexual changes I would like to see are the sexual discrimination acts rewritten, so sex is not defined whether you are a male or female, but sex is defined about sex in general. I think the current legislation should have been called the Gender Discrimination Act instead of the Sex Discrimination Act.

In the ACT [Australian Capital Territory] we have a more enlightened approach, which says you are not allowed to discriminate against someone on the basis of their occupation or their job. This was specifically introduced to stop people discriminating against sex workers and people who worked in the adult industry and to stop insurance companies, landlords and newspapers discriminating against them. If a sex worker goes to rent a flat and the landlord doesn't want to because of her job, this should be illegal. It is legal to do sex work in various states in Australia like the ACT, Victoria, New South Wales and

Queensland, but discrimination against individual workers continues.

It should be illegal to deny services and goods to people in the adult industry. Most politicians, no matter how liberal they were before they went into politics, believe they have to take a negative and restrictive approach to sexual regulation. In Melbourne it is illegal to advertise for staff, cleaners or receptionists for a brothel, because this is believed to be 'distasteful'. Most of the owners of tabletop dancing clubs and brothels are not sleaze bags and many of them are into spiritual awareness and New Age philosophies.

The texture of the sex industry has changed. It is now being run by more businesswomen and men who don't come from the sex industry, but other areas of retail and wholesaling. The men who were the traditional power brokers in the sex industry in the 1960s and 1970s are disappearing and a very different type of adult industry business is emerging. I feel middle management in the sex industry will be run by women in the next 10 years, as has already started to happen. The biggest growth area is in products for women, and this is reflected in the industry.

TIPS: Having a better sex life

To have a better sex life you need to broaden your awareness, and my advice is to learn to meditate. Do something that is unrelated to sex, expand your internal awareness and make yourself open to new thoughts. It might be psychoanalysis, astrology, meditation or an exercise programme. At the same time sit down with your partner and be really honest. Let's forget about the past, but from now on be totally honest about our sexual feelings to one another and other people. Small amounts of honesty beget bigger amounts of honesty because you know you have nothing to lose.

Speak your fantasies; it opens a new intimacy with your partner. If your partner closes down, and feels rejected, then the relationship has problems and at that point people have to be able to work on themselves. If the person doesn't like honesty then maybe the person has to work on their awareness. The reward is that you have better sex with your partner and you do not lose them. Trust is a wonderful turn-on; normally when you speak out your fantasies it doesn't go anywhere.

I have also found that being aware of the physiological changes that my body has gone through is helpful. For example, when I was younger I never thought that getting an erection would be an issue, and I am sure women going through menopause experience a lot of sexual changes that they never anticipated too.

I have noticed that over the past 10 years, from turning 40 to 50, that my orgasms have changed. They are much longer and I feel that the sensations continue five or 10 minutes after the event. I feel that if your life spirit is dim then your sexual spirit is dim.

5

All Kinds of People

'I'm exploring my sexual diversity' is one of those phrases that is easy to say, and that people generally accept, until they have to confront the reality. Non-traditional relating, whether it be an open relationship/marriage, an SM partnership, a *ménage à trois*, or sharing a kinky fantasy usually attracts either laughter, embarrassment or condemnation. Rarely is it seen as something that is positive to indulge in, something that can help people to grow and be valuable to a relationship.

Sexual diversity is widespread, yet ironically almost completely hidden. It is everywhere, but no one knows about it. Your next-door neighbour could well be a secret rubber fetishist, your member of parliament could be a bondage aficionado and your librarian may be an enthusiastic member of the local swingers' club.

The prevailing view is that people mate for life with one partner, have heterosexual sex in the missionary position, don't use sex toys, products or services – and yet somehow remain erotically fulfilled by this rather dull scenario. This widespread myth persists despite the fact that any cursory look through the phone directory, on the Internet, or in the back pages of your local paper disproves it.

Minority groups defined by their sexual difference usually do not have a public voice. It is only through spying specialist magazines, often on the top shelves of newsagents, or accidentally finding them on the Internet, that we discover their existence.

What is amazing is how often behind the outrageous façade the men in these different lifestyles yearn for love, acceptance and social recognition.

SM

Fantasies about sexually dominating someone, or being sexually submissive to someone, are very common but are often misunderstood. The essence of domination and submission is eroticised power and eroticised powerlessness, which can only be explored if you have a trusting relationship with your partner.

Erotic power play, or SM, is a sexual pivot around which many happy and healthy relationships revolve, as men in this chapter show. SM is about erotically submitting to your partner, or dominating them, with not only their full consent, but also their enthusiastic approval.

SM is usually portrayed as a violent, dangerous sexual activity and many people do not think there is any difference between a sadist, a masochist and a serial killer. However, an ethical concern for the people you sexually play with lies at the heart of SM and for any activity consent must not only be assumed but actively voiced. The misconceptions about SM make it hard for people involved in the scene to talk about their proclivities to others.

Within the SM scene the role of men is less understood than that of women, because a traditional Mistress archetype is so well known. This woman is usually resplendent in thigh-high boots with 6-inch heels, a tightly laced corset, a whip and a cruel expression – think Cruella de Ville meets Elvira, Mistress of the Dark.

The role of men in SM is less clear-cut. Most people have a vague image of a submissive man in bondage, or maybe infantilised in a nappy, but little idea how deep submissive fantasies go in the minds of many men. Sexually dominant men bring up mixed emotions for many women – what sort of man gets turned on by dominating a woman? Men involved in the SM lifestyle have a complex sexual path and in this chapter they explain how they integrate their sexuality into the rest of their life.

Swinging

The world of swingers is one where the old rules and conventions of marriage and monogamy have been overturned. It is where couples can live out their fantasies with other couples, and then retreat together back to their children, their suburban houses and their respectable jobs. For some it is liberating, the perfect synthesis of sexual freedom within a sexual commitment.

Swinging and open marriages came of age in the sixties, and many people's first view of the swinging lifestyle was the film *Bob & Carol & Ted & Alice*. It then seemed to die down, only to be currently undergoing a huge resurgence worldwide. Partner-swapping is now regarded as a 'lifestyle movement', not just a free love experiment.

Swingers' holiday resorts, clubs that cater to larger-sized swingers and swinger magazines are testament to the popularity of the movement. Swinging is widely regarded as the fastest growing area of sexuality. It is an area where each swinging couple can set their own boundaries, within the commitment to their marriage. For many swingers the lifestyle is seen as a hobby, a shared interest, something that binds them together. This is surprising to many people outside the swinging lifestyle, who see such 'sanctioned adultery' as the end of a happy partnership.

Layne Winklebleck

Layne Winklebleck was born in Portland, Oregon in 1938 and grew up in a rural community. In the 1970s he became a radical social worker, favouring encounter group work and gestalt therapy.

It was during this time that he accepted his SM fantasies, which had been part of his sexual life since adolescence. In 1979 he left his profession to expand his sexual horizons with his life partner, Kat

Sunlove. In San Francisco they staged SM productions with female dominance and male submission, as well as conducting workshops such as SM for Loving Couples.

They both started to write for The Berkeley Barb *magazine, which advocated sexual freedom and was sold to a mainstream audience through newsstands and vending machines. The articles and advertising in the magazine explored topless dancing, leather organisations, the sex industry and SM and fetish organisations and communities.*

Layne and Kat became so involved in the revolutionary approach that the magazine took that they bought it in the early 1980s, renaming it The Spectator. *They have successfully run the magazine since this time, supporting the views of sex workers, dominatrixes, adult video celebrities and erotic artists.*

Kat is presently a lobbyist for the Free Speech Coalition, a trade association for the adult entertainment industry, and Layne is the editor and general manager of The Spectator. *He feels that the importance and significance of the publication is its overarching vision of sexual tolerance and diversity.*

I was in the closet, in terms of my SM fantasies, until I was in my thirties, by which time I was a social work educator. I was influenced as a mental health professional during the seventies by the human encounter movement, Fritz Perls, psychodrama and the like. My radical approach led me to self-disclose about fantasies, become more and more open with everyone and gradually integrate my 'shadow side' into the rest of my being. I also came to an understanding of some of the emotional and quality of life costs we pay when we deny to ourselves or to others the truest nature of our sexual desires.

In the early seventies *The Berkeley Barb*, parent publication to *The Spectator* and a venerable counterculture publication of the 1960s, shone as a beacon of sexual freedom – even as far north as Seattle, where I languished in sexual purgatory, awaiting a better day. That day finally came in 1979 when I threw caution to the winds and joined my life partner, Kat Sunlove, in a most remarkable odyssey of sexual exploration (both hedonistic and intellectual) that has lasted to this day.

The topless dancing craze, the Summer of Love and other 1960s phenomena had identified San Francisco as a hotbed of sexual freedom. Sexual minorities of all kinds, yearning to breathe free, as it were, migrated there. *The Barb* (and later *The Spectator*) already represented libertarian values that we heartily endorsed when we arrived on the scene and played a well-known role in our history of sexual freedom. Our publication became a primary means for the sex community to do missionary outreach work, so to speak, and a way for people to find each other.

American society has become polarised regarding issues of freedom of sexual expression, with regional areas of tolerance on both coasts and in many urban centres, and in between an escalating intolerance for sexual expression in much of Middle America. Battles in this 'sex war' are fought on legal, adversarial grounds rather than through compromise and rational public debate.

Opinions tend to be absolutist and neither side will give an inch. In the short term a conservative administration and a conservative Supreme Court promise to make things hard on the good guys. Over the long haul, however, freedom will win the day because of the momentum of the media and the Internet. Intolerance and ignorance cannot survive in an atmosphere of open communication.

Real change has been happening at such a pace that I can hardly believe it. And everything is accelerating constantly. The pill, for goodness sake, is only 40 years old. How old is the Internet?

Classic SM is dominant woman/submissive man, with the man being the sexual object. However, when this changes, and the man becomes dominant and the woman submissive, many people criticise the scene as reflecting the traditional oppressive sex roles in our society.

I don't believe this is true, as the energies of SM play between players are basically the same, regardless of gender preferences. Experienced players almost universally recognise this and can enjoy the aesthetics and energy of a play scene based completely on the quality of the scene. A hot scene is a hot scene. I say, 'gender, schmender'.

Also, why worry about reflecting traditional oppressive gender roles? People can act out Nazi scenes, people do infantilism scenes. People do 'fetch the slippers for the Lord and Master' scenes. Whatever. Of course there are differences in an SM context, compared to actual historical gender roles. SM play is conscious rather than unconscious, consensual, loving, not actually traditional and not actually oppressive.

TIP: A secret tip from an SM Master/Switch

The energies of SM are intrapsychic, telepathic. The trick is to calibrate psychic energy so that both partners are on extreme opposite ends of a vortex of dominant/submissive emotion at the same time. There are many paths to this. I have learned, for example, how to replicate the special magic of this psychic joining with certain partners by using the give and take of oral-genital servitude as a platform.

The giver strives to truly and deeply believe, to hypnotise themselves and to let themselves truly become the total and absolute sex slave forever and never ever stopping, never tiring, never thinking of themselves unto death, with only love and trying to please, yes, yes, yes. You get the picture.

On the other end of the vortex of energy, the taker strives to truly believe, to hypnotise themselves and to truly become the total and absolute tyrant and taker. They do this without a care for their sex slave, with only their own selfish pleasure as an objective, forever and ever, as long as they may wish to bask in pleasure.

That's the other side of the picture. Behaviours are not enough. In fact, if you can reach these places in the mind without them, behaviours are not even necessary. How many partners have I proved this to? How many amazed looks when finally she let her mind go to the place I had asked her for and felt the magic? Ah, yes. Those were the good old days.

Of course I realise many readers will roll their eyes at this. Most folks have not incorporated the idea of intrapsychic energies into their belief systems. Try this exercise, because even if only one couple tries and succeeds in this path to the true magic, the sum addition of total pleasure to the universe will be well worth it.

Robert McGinley

Dr Robert McGinley was born in Los Angeles and has lived in New Jersey, Delaware and Japan. He is the founder and president of one of the most unique companies in the world, The Lifestyles Organization, also known simply as Lifestyles. It sponsors the oldest (26 years) and largest (4,000 attendees) annual Lifestyles Convention, with people from across the US and over 20 other countries coming together for three or more days and nights of social intimacy, sensual fun and educational opportunities.

The Lifestyles Sensual & Erotic Art Exhibit, often featuring art that has been censored in other times and places, is now a highly regarded institution within the international art community. Lifestyles also offers monthly sensual dinner dances for couples, along with Valentine, Mardi Gras, Hallowe'en and New Year's Eve balls.

Robert is also co-director and co-founder of Club WideWorld, one of America's longest continuously operated, private membership swing clubs for couples. He is the chairman and CEO of Lifestyles Tours & Travel, the US's first full service travel agency that started, and now specialises in, exotic, lifestyle-oriented couples' tours.

He is the founder/president of NASCA International, an association of clubs, publications and individuals in the swing community. He has written numerous articles on swinging, relationships, society and sexuality. He has appeared on many of America's top television talk shows, including The Phil Donahue Show, Hour Magazine, Chicago AM, People Are Talking, Sally Jessy Raphael *and* Geraldo *and many radio talk programmes.*

He has been interviewed by USA Today, *the* Los Angeles Times, The Register, Forum, Time, Penthouse, Stern *and many other publications. He is known in North America, Europe and Japan as a lifestyles and personal freedom activist. Robert is listed in* How I Got Into Sex *by Drs Bonnie & Vern Bullough, William Hartman, Marilyn Fithian and Randy Sue Klein and his life and work is presented in* The Lifestyle: A Look at the Erotic Rites of Swingers *by Terry Gould. His hobbies include the preservation of WWII aircraft, photography and travel. He holds an MA and a Ph.D. in Counselling Psychology. He has been married twice, has five children and lives in California.*

I have been interested in sex since puberty and became interested in swingers, though it was not called that then, in Japan in 1967. When I returned to Berkeley, California I became involved with the Sexual Freedom Link, which no longer exists. It was not a swinging group but a political activist organisation and was very singles orientated. I was divorced at that time and the discussions were with mostly divorced men and women.

This group became very sexual and turned into the Club WideWorld, where I met my girlfriend, who later became my wife. This has grown to be a corporation known as LSO and still has a swing club, but also has a Lifestyles Convention, Tours & Travel, NASCA International and Europa [covering all of Europe]. We have been busy organising swing clubs in Europe, especially Germany. Although there are more swing clubs in Northern America than the rest of the world, there are swing clubs in every Western country.

Swinging is now an economic force because there are clubs and conventions where people spend a great deal of money. For example, we have a tour in Jamaica of 1,000 people who spend about US $1,000 per person. So it has become an economic force far beyond the sexual connotations.

Swinging has grown in popularity worldwide. It is primarily a social activity of couples, but some swing clubs do admit singles, primarily single men. Swinging has also become more accepted by mainstream society. The lifestyle transcends national borders, race and even age. It has become a way to bring people together.

This is not an activity for all people but the couples involved are predominantly middle to upper middle class. The age is mid-20s to the mid-50s. Their relationships are very honest, with a lot of respect without a power struggle. They are people who have a good opinion of themselves and are not easily threatened by jealousy.

There are some people who try swinging and it doesn't work for them. There is not much swinging in the Latin American countries, or highly religious societies, because they are governed by a lot of guilt.

For a couple to go to a swing club they would have had to already discuss the issues between themselves first. This is not common in most marriages, because most people would not dare to voice their fantasies and desires about having sex with someone else.

Swinging attracts couples that already 'have it together'. In a sense, the lifestyle/social recreation attracts 'the cream of the crop' of couples. They don't generally become swingers to spice up their life; rather, swinging is a natural path of couples already enjoying their life. Their openness to communicate to each other about this is carried on in their relationships with others. The couples involved have a clear understanding of what is sex and what is love. They use sex for recreation and relaxation, whereas many people mix up the two, thinking if you have sex with someone you have to fall in love with them.

Before the Internet it was much more difficult to find people who were interested in swinging. Now with online chat sites and sex sites the whole area has opened up. Viagra has also changed things and generated discussion and openness about sex and sexual issues.

The down side to swinging is not the activity, but the people involved. For some people their religious beliefs cause them to feel guilty after participating in such activity, while other times it doesn't work because the man has pressured his partner to go along.

My answer to world peace is to turn the United Nations into a swinging club, because you wouldn't want to drop a bomb on someone you just had an orgasm with.

TIP: What to expect at a swing club

If it is your first time at a swingers' event it is important to interview the organisers of the club or party you want to go to. Initially you might like to go to a swinging dance, which is a non-sexual party.

For couples it is important that before they go to a swinging activity they are open and honest with one another, and talk about anything they may feel uncomfortable about. Good communication is essential, and because of that most couples that become involved with swinging experience little jealousy. As there are no written rules to swinging you should not set rules for one another.

Swing clubs and parties do differ depending on what country they are in. Over the years many swinging activities have moved away from sexual activity to a more social one. Some swinging activities are a dance where there is no open sex at all and there is a bit of feeling up on the dancefloor. A couple might meet another couple and go to a hotel room.

Often at a swing club they have rooms set aside specifically for sexual activity. Some will be private and some will be a group room with many couples on beds pushed together.

6

That's the Way Sex Is

For most of us, sex is not something that we would spend a whole day or evening preparing for, but in many ancient cultures this was an accepted practice. Time was put aside to explore the sensuality of the body and expand pleasure, as people believed there was a strong link between spirituality, sex, health and longevity.

The concept of spiritual or sacred sexuality originally came from the rituals of the Sumerian goddess of love and sexuality, Inanna, and Ishtar, the Babylonian goddess of love and war, from ancient Chinese Taoist practices and Indian tantric philosophy.

Several sexology classics have become the basis of the art of making love. *The Elemental Maid*, written in the 1st century AD in China, suggests that good health comes from good sex. India has the Hindu scriptures of the *Kama Sutra*, written during the 3rd and 4th centuries AD, while Japan had a sex manual called *Shunga*. Both of these expanded lovemaking positions. In the Middle East there was the Arabic *Tales of the Perfumed Garden*, written in the 14th and 15th centuries.

These cultures realised the significance of lovemaking techniques that were an essential way to develop spiritually or make a religious connection with the divine. On a more mundane level they were a way to prolong pleasure and help fulfil a relationship.

All the teachings emphasised that it was beneficial for men to delay or refrain from ejaculation, and encouraged women to orgasm. To achieve this they drew on an array of techniques taken from meditation, breathing, visualisation, yogic positions and erotic ritual, whose central tenet is the weaving of the masculine and feminine energy that is in each of us.

Visual images have been used for centuries to celebrate and externalise the erotic. With the invention of the camera a new visual erotic arena opened up. It is often assumed that men are only interested in, and aroused by, graphic depictions of sex, described by many women as 'just gynaecology shots' or 'huge dicks taking up the screen'. However, many men seek out sensual, erotic images, finding inspiration from nature and images that allow them to be involved with the subject.

It is not just women who have wholeheartedly embraced the early Eastern sexual practices. Tantric and Taoist sex is enthusiastically followed by many of the men in this chapter, who have found its holistic view of male sexuality to be wonderfully refreshing and emotionally fulfilling.

Erotic genital massage has been taught by men in the West for a number of years and brings ancient wisdom to the modern world. Its popularity expanded during the 1980s when people's fear of intimacy was being exacerbated by the worldwide panic over HIV/AIDS. It was seen then as a way to keep sexuality alive in a sex-negative time of near hysteria about the virus.

The massage has retained its popularity, as it is a great alternative to traditional sex, or an accompaniment to it. It allows couples to go deeper into sexual pleasure and provides a new way to enjoy sex without pressure or anxieties about performance.

Many men have found that whole new areas of their sexuality have opened up when embracing tantric and Taoist styles of sensuality, and this has led them to question the limited and limiting ways in which men are allowed to express their sexuality in the West.

In the Eastern techniques men have to learn to give up control, to let themselves surrender to pleasure and this type of intimacy, but loss of control is traditionally seen as effeminate (being 'like a woman'). Men have been taught to be contemptuous of 'soft' sexual behaviour, such as massage and intimate touch, to their own detriment.

Teaching men that they must always be in sexual (and emotional) control is a prescription for emotional and sexual dysfunction. The men in this chapter show that the ability to give up sexual control, to let go, is at the heart of the best and most profound orgasmic sexual experiences.

David Steinberg

David Steinberg lives in Santa Cruz, USA. He is an author, editor and publisher of artistic, imaginative sexual and erotic material, intended as an alternative to commercial pornography. His books include Erotic by Nature: A Celebration of Life, of Love and of Our Wonderful Bodies; The Erotic Impulse: Honouring the Sensual Self; Father Journal: Five Years of Awakening to Fatherhood; Beneath This Calm Exterior *(poems) and* Yellow Brick Road: Steps Toward a New Way of Life.

He is the co-creator and producer of Celebration of Eros, *a multimedia erotic theatre presentation; associate editor of* Sexuality and Culture *magazine; contributing writer and columnist for* The Spectator *magazine and US photo representative for* Cupido *magazine (Norway/Denmark).*

His writing has appeared in such journals as Salon, Playboy, Boston Phoenix, Los Angeles Weekly, San Jose Metro, Sexuality and Culture, Spectator, Cupido, The Sun, Libido, The Realist, CleanSheets, Scarlet Letters, JaneZine, Mothering, Journal of Gender Studies, Learning, Commonweal, Gauntlet, Changing Men *and* Issues in Radical Therapy.

He is currently completing a book of his essays, This Thing We Call Sex: Reflections on the Culture and Politics of Sex in America *and editing a second book of erotic photography,* Sex Is: Sexual Photography Comes of Age.

I began writing about sex in the late 1980s. I was active in the feminist community, where discussion of pornography was quite active. A number of us felt that it was important to do more in response to pornography than criticise it, that if we didn't like the ways that women, men and sex were portrayed in porn, we should come up with something better of our own. With a close woman friend, I began to collect material for what we thought would be an alternative erotic journal, but turned instead into a book of erotic and sexual photography and fiction, *Erotic by Nature: A Celebration of Life, of Love and of Our Wonderful Bodies*, which was published in 1988. The book quickly became very popular and threw me into the world of people doing intelligent writing, thinking and publishing about sex, many of them in the San Francisco area.

The fundamental issue that I keep coming back to in my writing, and now in my photography as well, is the importance of enthusiastically embracing our sexual natures, even (or especially) when those natures ache to express themselves in ways that run across the grain of approved social/sexual mores.

Christian culture treats sex as a danger and a problem rather than as a source of pleasure, personal fulfilment and wisdom. We need to understand what we're up against culturally, and be willing to follow and develop our sexual natures rather than fear and repress them.

Personally, I've found that my sexual tastes and interests change over time and rarely stay within the bounds of what society considers proper or acceptable. All of my writing and photography goes back to my personal experience. Even though my lifestyle is more oriented to my sexuality than most people's, I feel that whatever is going on inside of me sexually is probably going on inside lots of other people as well, even if they may be reluctant to admit it to themselves. So I take off from what I feel and have found that I often strike chords that resonate strongly in a broad spectrum of other people.

I think I can talk better about a 'good erotic photograph' than a 'good erotic photographer'. Let's say that a 'good erotic photographer' is someone who takes 'good erotic photographs'. For me, an erotic photograph (or more specifically, a sexual photograph) is successful if it causes the viewer to think about sex in a new way, in a way that goes beyond the narrow stereotypes of 'what is sexy' that mainstream culture puts out. I like photos that encourage people to explore new areas of their own sexual feelings, and that encourage them to think of sex more broadly than how pretty, young, thin, heterosexual people have intercourse.

I am editing a book of sexual photography now that will be a statement about both photography and sex – hopefully broadening readers' thinking about both. It will include kissing and touching and dancing as well as fucking and sucking, heavy people as well as thin people, old people as well as young, disabled people as well as able-bodied people. We all tend to live in about 1 per cent of the sexual spectrum available to us, which seems very sad and limiting to me.

Right now I am really consumed by the photo project I have taken on, trying to capture something real and compelling about people having sex on film. The issue, to me, is largely about intimacy, vulnerability, the subtlety of intense passion and love. I think we have all had our fill of pretence and various versions of supposedly 'super sex'. In the end, I suspect the most fulfilling sex for most people comes down to some very simple things: vulnerability, connection, getting outside one's own skin, feeling loved and loving, breaking through the loneliness inherent in being physically separate from every other person.

TIP: Taking erotic photos of your lover

For me, the most powerful pictures are the ones where the people are most real. This is where they reveal something of themselves not often seen on film, though maybe often seen by their partner during sex. A lot has to do with people not feeling self-conscious in front of the camera, unless it's someone who just loves to be in front of the camera, which is something else altogether. Taking photos can be fun in itself, and if you're both having fun, you'll probably get great pictures.

Smiles and playfulness photograph much better than people think, while 'ooh-baby' intense looks most often come off as looking like every stock porn picture you've ever seen (though there are some notable exceptions). I would say just try to be honest and don't try too hard; follow the energy generated by the presence of the camera rather than trying to lead it around by the nose.

Kenneth Ray Stubbs

Kenneth Ray Stubbs is a sociologist with a Ph.D. in psychology/holistic health sciences and is a certified sex educator and sexologist. He has trained in numerous areas of sexuality, including tantric and Taoist practices, and has studied Buddhism, meditation, t'ai chi ch'uan, shiatsu, polarity therapy and massage.

Since 1981 he has been the editor and owner of Secret Garden Publishing. He is the author of nine titles on sexuality, including Erotic Passions, The Essential Tantra, Secret Sexual Positions, Male Erotic Massage, The Clitoral Kiss *and* Erotic Massage. *He has contributed to* How I Got Interested in Sex *by Dr Bonnie Bullough and to computer magazines. He was a columnist for the German edition of* Penthouse *and has also produced the video* Erotic Massage. *He is currently working on his new book,* Kiss of Desire.

He lives in the Sonoran Desert near Tucson, Arizona.

There are no temples, no tradition or teachers, we are all learning about tantra and sacred sexuality by the seat of our pants. It is a very different world from that of the tantric beginnings, which were 1,700 to 1,800 years ago in ancient India. It's a struggle to find what to do and how to be, to look at sexuality from a different perspective than what society projects.

I feel learning, teaching and writing about sexuality has been my destiny. I grew up in a southern Baptist family, which was very stable and loving. I did not come from a sexual abuse background other than the sexual negativity of the Church. I had to work past this indoctrination and I feel it's something that we all have to do. At 17 years of age I decided my only option was to become an atheist, to escape the Church's oppressive dogma.

It was 1968, the counter-cultural revolution was in full bloom, and the image of what female sexuality was was blown asunder in the hippie culture. I was an assistant at a planned parenthood clinic in Chicago which had a very sex-positive view.

This influenced me many years later to learn about tantra and spiritual sexuality. I studied with a lama in Berkeley at the Tibetan Buddhist Centre for nine months, learning meditation, yoga and how to expand my body energy. I was also at the time teaching erotic massage and would go from one extreme to another, from five- to six-day retreats in silence with no touching and sexual expression, to exactly the opposite.

I had been a sociologist, and studied erotic massage and taught it because I felt sexual energy had been excluded in our society. It was part of an oppressive indoctrination that the genitals were off-limits. I was so at home with the touch of the body that I started integrating it with the energy experiences I had been having, and realised that this was the essence of the Buddhist teaching of mindfulness. Meditation is about being here now; mindfulness is the key and the essence of tantra.

If I were teaching Love Making 1 to beginners, I would teach sensual massage, focusing on long, slow, sensual touch. All aspects of lovemaking can transfer over from this, be it oral, intercourse or an erotic movement. It is also important for people to get touched. Being a good lover is about taking time. Its essence is relaxing and letting things unfold, feeling and having permission to touch, kiss, insert, embrace.

I had a neck injury when I was 46 years old, which came about from a sexual energy experience. I had been working for many years on expanding my orgasmic energy through meditation and yoga, and one day had an orgasm that was so intense that my body couldn't stand it. I fell and hurt myself severely, injuring a ligament in my neck.

The main way that I made love before the accident was with my hands, but the sensations in my hands have not come back. Other areas of my body have sensations of about 50 to 80 per cent what they were before the accident. As a result I can't be a lover like I was before. I can have erections, but the sensation is not the same, so now I concentrate on having energy orgasms. I now focus on meditation and my energy pattern, but I am grateful that I can still write.

The cutting edge of my growth has been orgasmic energy and this led me to write about sacred orgasms in my book *Essential Tantra*. I saw the link between spirituality and sexuality. When I learnt about massage I learnt about energy. I did not want to focus on orgasms; for 10 years I played with expanding orgasmic energy. This led on to my meditation and chakra study.

There are four types of orgasmic systems that connect with chakras or energy centres throughout the body. These are not necessarily sexual, or orgasmic, but they can occur in conjunction with sexual energy streaming through the body. The sensations can feel like a rocket ship exploding. The things that helped me expand my sexual sensations were deep body massage, masturbation and meditation; through these I was able to experience full-body orgasm, which is available to all of us.

EXERCISE: THE TIGER'S KISS

This must be done with care and sensitivity to keep your partner coming back for more. Depending on his or her level of arousal, the same bite might elicit either anger or intense passion.

Arouse your lover with sensual touch, focusing on the area at the back of the neck. At the side of the spine there are two long muscles – lick, kiss, suck and gently bite the area of one side. Locate a thick and perhaps tight muscle, maybe along the upper shoulder or the back of the neck. Slowly bite into the muscle until you sense your lover is at the edge of pain, then bite a tiny bit more. Hold for a fleeting moment, or if your lover is moaning with pleasure, for a couple of seconds, before releasing.

Kerry Riley

Kerry Riley was born in Newcastle, Australia and grew up in the 1970s. After completing a degree in psychology and mathematics his first job was in industrial mathematics. He then taught maths at a boys' school. At the age of 26 he wanted to explore more and spent two years travelling the world.

In the East he came across teachings relating to the development of mind, body and spirit. He was amazed to discover that some spiritual practices not only included sex but also revered the study of sensual loving, seeing it as sacred. On returning to Australia he met and married Diane, a woman with a similar background and desire for personal exploration and growth.

Kerry started to teach yoga and meditation, and to practise acupuncture and Chinese medicine. He developed a highly successful course on personal empowerment called 'Mindpowers', which thousands of people attended. He and Diane developed several courses on love, sex and relationships, from beginner to advanced levels.

After one of their workshops, a week-long retreat, the couple was blessed with an awesomely magical lovemaking experience. It was so powerful that for the next 15 years they explored the great traditions of ecstatic sexuality, including Taoist sexology from ancient China and tantra from ancient India, shaman Indian sexuality from North America and sacred women's sexuality from ancient Babylon. They combined these secrets and practices with the most recent research on sexuality from universities and sex therapists throughout the world, and read and studied extensively with numerous authors and teachers in this field.

Kerry has an extensive background in the human potential area. He has lectured to more than 40,000 people and produced numerous programmes on video and cassette. Together with Diane he was featured in the film Secrets of Sacred Sex – A Guide to Love and Intimacy, *which was acclaimed worldwide. They are the authors of the bestselling book* Sexual Secrets for Men – What Every Woman Will Want Her Man to Know, *and conduct practical programmes in relationships and sensual loving.*

Their most recent work provides men with a unique experience in tantra. Private lessons can be arranged with a tantric goddess skilled in the arts of love and sensuality.

Kerry and Diane Riley live on the northern beaches of Sydney. Besides teaching tantra, Kerry enjoys surfing, which he does almost every day, salsa dancing, family life with his three children, Soelae, Lisa and Sam, and most of all making love with Diane.

Sex has always been of central importance [to me]. When I was younger it preoccupied my mind and every time I met a woman I'd be thinking about the possibility of getting into bed with her. When I met my wife Diane we made love practically every day and sex was something that took us into a beautiful connected space. Through our sexual loving I felt closer than I felt to any other human being. When we met, both Diane and I were involved in yoga and meditation to find a deeper meaning in life, and in searching many teachings for a way of life that spoke to us on a spiritual level. But we also loved the raw, sexual, physical sensations of having sex. Our discovery of tantric sex was a true blessing because it showed us a way of connecting our sexuality with our spirituality. It gave us three important ideas:

1. How to turn sex into making love;
2. Pleasure into ecstasy;
3. Partnership into union.

These three elements have been the cornerstone to our 20-year relationship. Sexuality is the juice that allows us to keep magic happening in our lives together and is why sexuality has been, and still is, so important to us both.

As a child I was taught, as I am sure many people were, that the way to God was through prayer and going to church. However, these things never gave me any profound experience of God. Through sexual union with my beloved I have a tangible experience of the divine or God, or the Goddess, or whatever one wants to call it. I have touched spaces of feeling a deep connectedness, not only to my beloved but to the whole cosmos. Precious moments of deep love and states of higher consciousness. When it happens like that it is magic, it is a doorway to enlightenment. I find it far more spiritual than going to church.

In my twenties I spent two years in Asia, mostly in India. The last six months away I was really sick with a tropical illness and I was exhausted. When I arrived back in Australia I had an interest in sex, but couldn't make love more than once a week without feeling exhausted. I had lost my Chi. As a young man so connected to his sexuality, I was devastated. It took me to the edge.

It was only through the teaching and practices of the ancient Chinese Taoist sexologists that I regained my drive. I learnt the secrets of ejaculation control and ways to make love over and over again without physical loss of energy. It taught me what every young man dreams about: being able to make love for as long as he likes, confident he is able to keep up with the physical needs of any woman. Of course I discovered later and know well now that lovemaking isn't just how you perform, how many strokes you can do; it is how much love you can send to your partner through your wand of light that really counts.

Something that really turned my life around was an experience I had with Diane. It happened after a week-long workshop we were conducting called 'Awakening Another Reality', which worked on opening people up to new dimensions physically, emotionally and spiritually. We had been away in the bush for two weeks. When we returned home we were at a very high level of consciousness. Diane and I created a lovemaking session that had all the elements of ceremony. Although we knew nothing of such rituals at the time, it just naturally happened. After about two hours Diane's whole face changed. I have never seen her looking so beautiful. She said to me, 'Your eyes are golden.' She literally saw my eyes as gold. She was seeing something beyond me and it felt so wonderful, beyond this earth entirely. After that there was a period in timelessness and no thought. We woke up stunned by the experience and were more deeply in love than ever before. We didn't tell anybody about it for many years until we read about a tantric experience almost exactly the same as our own. To us this extraordinary experience was a gift, and a clear message to seek this path further in our lives, and we both felt blessed.

It is said in tantric writings that when a couple is in sexual bliss the angels of love come and dance on the ceiling, and Shaktia and Shiva take on human form. Whatever happened it touched our lives for ever and was an inspiration that made us want to share it with others. Sacred sex became not only our interest but our profession. We did the video, *Secrets of Sacred Sex: A Guide to Love and Intimacy*, which sold over 200,000 copies worldwide and we wrote a great book, *Sexual Secrets for Men: What Every Woman Will Want Her Man to Know*, which has helped and continues to help thousands of people on their journey into love.

Men can learn to open their hearts so that during lovemaking they are feeling as much energy in their heart as they are in their genitals. Then sex becomes lovemaking and that's a big difference. Second, they can learn the skills of ejaculation control, to be able to make love over and over again or at least as long as they want to. Long enough to feel the love that is happening, rather than concentrating on his or her orgasm. Third, they can learn to experience whole body orgasm rather than love ejaculation. Fourth, they can learn to create a sacred experience with their lovemaking, one that will touch them and their partner on every level: body, heart and soul.

These are some of the skills of tantra. Our video and workshops teach these skills; however, what really counts is having the experience. But how do you get the experience? At my men's seminars, men would often express a concern that they didn't have anyone to practise with, they were not confident about trying some of these practices with a new lover or their partner wasn't interested. Through Diane's women's workshops, she has connections with some single women who were skilled in the arts of tantra and who were willing to guide in the practices of sacred love. This was only for men who authentically wanted to learn and who were willing to meet these women first to see if there was a mutual attraction.

In ancient times there were women who lived in the temples of Aphrodite, the goddess of love and sensuality. They were the temple priestesses, who would use their lovemaking skills for healing and transformation, to give a man a tangible experience of the love of the goddess Aphrodite and a connection to the sacred.

There is no better way to learn tantra than with a woman experienced in the arts of the goddess. A client, Scott, who had studied with me, related this story after a couple of sessions with Jasmine, who had been trained in the arts of tantra and Taoist techniques. He said, 'I felt completely nurtured and pampered in the arms of the goddess. I experienced that I could handle higher levels of pleasure without fear of ejaculating too soon. I trusted her enough to open my heart and she helped me verbalise my feelings. It was an invaluable practice in ways of giving a woman greater pleasure, both physically and emotionally. It was a relief to be able to ask questions and get guidance without being put down like had happened to me previously. My marriage of eight years was difficult for the last three years. My wife was always criticising me for not lasting long enough. Sex was hardly happening between us. After our break-up, whenever I met a new woman I would find myself avoiding getting too intimate with her in case she discovered I wasn't the best lover. Recently I met a lady I really liked and even though I read about tantra I found myself not game to introduce her to it; I guess I was afraid. However, now that I have had the practice with Jasmine I feel so much more confident about trying it with others. It has been an extremely valuable experience for me.'

By having an experience of a woman skilled in the arts of the temple priestess a man clearly gets to see that he can develop to be a far better lover.

Exercises – How to keep the sparkle in your sex life

There are a lot of people that don't even try to spice up their sex life. They just go along with their lives and expect their love life will look after itself. Career, money, family and kids become their main concerns. Then they wonder why their partner cheated or why there is no passion like before. I know you love your partner, but are you 'in love' with them? Other couples realise after a few years that they are losing that 'in love' passionate sex and they seek help, which can be marriage counsellors, books, videos, romantic holidays, sexual-enhancing performance drugs, threesomes. All can help – different couples use different things at different stages of their relationship.

Many couples that consult us know what they should do but their modern busy lifestyle gets in the way of their good intentions. There are two exercises we have found that get the best results in the long term. I think one of the main reasons that they work is that they are simple, they don't take long.

Exercise 1

This is an appreciation exercise. One of the problems of marriage is that often each of us feels that we are not being appreciated for what we do. This is because we forget to voice our appreciation of love. Commonly we do not realise that we get into the habit of finding what our partner does wrong. We need to make it a daily practice to scan all the things they do and find something they are doing 'right', and tell them how much we enjoy it. When was the last time you told your beloved that you really appreciate the meals they cook? That you think he or she is doing a great job with the kids and you really appreciate them organising social events. During the next couple of days, whenever your partner gives you a suggestion about something, try saying, 'That's a great idea'. Even though you may not intend to take action, at least give them some acknowledgement, say, 'That is a great idea, thanks for that, I will consider it!', or the next time she does something that she perhaps does every day, such as preparing the meals, say to her, 'I really appreciate the cooked dinner'.

So often a man takes it for granted that his partner knows he appreciates what she does. Women also often take it for granted that the man knows he is appreciated. Sometimes a woman won't say something because she is still angry about all the things he does that she doesn't like. Because she never acknowledges him why should he acknowledge her? It grows into a competition for power. As teammates in love we should be empowering each other to feel good, but instead we often get into the habit of fault finding and then only empower each other to feel bad.

EXERCISE 2

Take five minutes out of your day, away from kids and everything else, sit opposite each other, hold hands, put some heart-touching background music on, close your eyes and for a minute start thinking about all the things that you appreciate about your partner. Open your eyes and then take turns in sharing five things you appreciate. You say five, your partner simply says, 'Thank you', then they say five. Repeat it, another five things each, and let this go on for a period of up to five minutes.

This is a very powerful exercise but it is almost a waste of time reading it without doing it. It is so simple you may think it won't make a difference. Do it for a week, see what happens. A lot of men might think this has got nothing to do with spicing up their sex life. That is where they are wrong. It has everything to do with it, as you will discover. Try it for one week soon.

7

Sexual Healing

The study of men's sexual health has traditionally seen men as a series of parts, some of which may have malfunctioned and need to be put right. Fear and misconceptions still surround most of men's sexual concerns, compounded by the fact that often men know little about their bodies, or the physical and psychological basis for their sexual problems and issues.

They often fall into the trap of seeing themselves as just the sum of 'parts', without knowing that a holistic view of their health is essential. The women's health movement of the 1970s revolutionised ideas about female health, but the equivalent for men, although sorely needed, has been slow in coming.

One of the original impetuses for this book was to highlight to women and men the variety of sexual writers and healers now working in the area of men's sexuality. I have worked in the equivalent area for women and often they have asked me whether there are radical healers working with men. In the past my answer has regrettably been 'No'. Now male sexual healers, from traditional and alternative schools of medicine and healing, are coming into their own.

No matter how informed male doctors and healers are, they have been confronted with the fact that their male clients are often still labouring under fundamental misconceptions about their own bodies, and particularly their own sexuality.

Male sexual healers see that men only have an adolescent model of male sexuality available to them. This model says that:

- sex is a performance that men must orchestrate;
- men always want sex and are always ready to 'get at it';
- sex requires an erection and always leads to intercourse;
- all physical contact must lead to sex;
- good sex is defined as increasing excitement that always ends in orgasm and ejaculation;
- all sexual contact must lead to sex;

- sex should 'just happen' and when it does men will 'naturally' know what to do.

The writers and sexual educators say that rather than spontaneously having great sex, with bodies that never let them down, most men are beset with concerns about their penis size and their sexual performance. One of the medical journalists in this chapter urges men to make peace with their penis and to turn off to, rather than turn on to, ideas about putting on a great sexual performance.

While post-menopausal women are throwing out old ideas of themselves as 'no longer interested in sex', so older men need new views of what constitutes an ageing, but still vital, sexuality. Often in mid-life men's sexuality is undergoing challenges, while women are coming into their own power.

At the moment the only discussion of older men and sexuality is a short one. It is summed up in a single word – Viagra. Viagra is often seen as a miracle drug, the answer to all of men's sexual and performance problems, so much so that it is one of the legal pharmaceuticals, like Valium, that has entered the vocabulary of stand-up comics and pop psychology. Take Viagra, buy a red sports car or a Harley Davidson motorbike, run off with a blonde 21-year-old – the Hollywood way to deal with the normal sexual changes that happen when a man ages.

Many far-thinking sex activists see great danger in this approach because it reverts men to a teenage model of sexuality where sexual prowess was measured by the length and hardness of an erection. It leaves unanswered the questions 'What is prowess?' and 'What makes a man feel sexually whole and good about himself?', and again sets a man at war with his penis.

While men seem to talk a lot about sex, it seems they are talking to the wrong people. An interesting statistic I came across while researching this book showed that in every typical consultation with a doctor a woman asks four questions and a man asks none.

Men need to talk more about sex and have more meaningful discussions. A frightening statistic in 2000 showed that in Western countries two thirds of the new cases of sexually transmitted diseases each year occur in people under 25. A quarter of these are in teenagers and most infections occur directly because of lack of knowledge.

There are wonderful new information sources available online, free and ensuring anonymity. Many of the writers profiled in this chapter are regular contributors to Web-based health services for men. This is a great way to access the best new thinking on male sexuality, and read material on areas that may be confronting and therefore difficult to seek out, such as male/male sexual abuse.

When asked if he could give one piece of advice to men, one of the contributors to this chapter urged that men heal the heart–genital connection, and change their sexual ethos from 'scoring' to 'caring'.

Dr Jules Black

Dr Jules Black was born and brought up in Sydney and has been an obstetrician and gynaecologist for 30 years, with a sub-speciality in the management of female and male sexual dysfunctions. A Fellow of the Royal College of Obstetricians & Gynaecologists and a Fellow of the Royal Australian & New Zealand College of Obstetricians & Gynaecologists, he is Australia's foremost gynaecological sexologist. In 1974 he was the first doctor to publish an article in the Australian and New Zealand Journal of Obstetrics and Gynaecology *drawing his fellow professionals' attention to their responsibility to help and educate their patients about sexuality and sexual needs.*

He has specialised in orgasmic dysfunctions and dyspareunia (painful intercourse in women). He is well-known for his speciality, which is helping women with vaginismus, the difficulty of consummating a sexual relationship, caused by the involuntary spasm of the pelvic floor muscles surrounding the vaginal introitus. It is largely associated with an overwhelming penetration anxiety, which in turn is due to multiple factors.

He has written BodyTalk: An A to Z Guide to Women's Health, *as well as numerous professional papers, book chapters and articles in medical and non-medical magazines and books. He is committed to all aspects of sex education, which he believes should be for everyone, and has often appeared in the media in this capacity.*

He has lectured at medical schools around the world, and given workshops and presented papers at domestic and international conferences. Since 1978 he has been a member of both the British Association of Sexual and Marital Therapy (BASMT) and the Society for Scientific Study of Sexuality (SSSS), serving as the latter's International Board Representative between 1983 and 1991.

Since 1985 he has been a board member of the World Association for Sexology (WAS), and served as its Secretary-General/Treasurer from 1989 to 1993. Since 1978 he has been an associate member of the International Academy of Sex Research (IASR). He lives in Sydney, Australia and has two daughters.

In the 1970s I was one of the pioneers in Australia in the area of sexuality. I had always felt that the sexuality of our patients is important, but it wasn't taught in medical school. We learnt about pregnancy and its physiology, biochemistry, endocrinology and anatomy, but that was all. In psychiatry we learnt about Freudian analysis, but never about the sexual act itself.

Nowhere did we learn about the very act on which our speciality depends, as in traditional medical education there appears to be no sex in pregnancy, sexually transmitted diseases, or birth control. I thought this was wrong and I decided that this area of sexuality is what I would specialise in.

On my first night as a doctor I was 23 years old and stationed in a large teaching hospital. I thought I might get someone coming in with a really rare disease, but instead a woman came in and told me that she had never had an orgasm. I discovered no one listens to a junior resident, or even a senior resident, so I realised I had to become a specialist before the medical establishment would listen to me. Once I became specialised my opinion was valued.

Recently I was doing a locum in a country hospital and a woman came in with intermittent pelvic pain. I asked the resident to ask her if she had ever had an orgasm, because the symptoms sounded very much like pelvic congestion. We got busy and I was summoned to the theatre by the surgeon before seeing the resident again. The surgeon called me up to have a peek and to give a gynaecological opinion. Her pelvis was clean, with no infection.

All her organs were fine, until the other doctor pointed out her right ovary, which had huge veins all over it. I took one look at it and said, 'This woman has never had an orgasm. This is classic Pelvic Congestion Syndrome.' (My resident told me afterwards that the woman had not had sex for over three and a half years.) The other surgeon could not cope at all with my comments but I was not surprised that doctors still can't handle talking about sex.

Most gynaecologists also still have a problem with this area. I will often come into the car park and see colleagues and they will ask, 'Are you still doing that...' and they often can't even say the words 'sex therapy'. I say I find it impossible to divorce the sexual act from my gynaecology work and they reply, 'I do my best to'.

I saw a woman recently in hospital who had a vaginal hysterectomy and her doctor hadn't talked to her about when she could resume sex. When I asked why she hadn't raised the issue she said he was such a nice man that she couldn't talk about sex [with him]. Many doctors give their patients the message that they do not want to be asked about sex, whereas my own patients see I am comfortable with the subject and can talk to me about orgasms, sex and any problems they have.

Many women perceive that a lot of my colleagues don't actually like women and it comes across when they interact with their clients. I feel their wives are often in part responsible because they are very negative about their husbands' patients, feeling that women interfere with their private lives. This attitude then rubs off on their husbands.

My work in the area of sexology has affected me negatively in my profession and the climb up the corporate ladder. People in my position all over the world find that this happens. Those in positions of power in hospitals have effectively blocked our promotions because of our stated interest in sexuality.

There was a president of the [now closed] Crown Street Women's Hospital, who was also president of a bank, who said that he had seen in the hospital's library a magazine article about a woman having sex with a dog, so he immediately ordered the removal of the magazine. This is the sort of thing I have had to face throughout my career. I told him I put that article in there and it was abstracted from the *American Journal of Obstetrics and Gynecology*, which is one of the most prestigious OB/GYN journals in the world. It was a case about a heavily pregnant woman whose man had left her and she was feeling extremely sexual, so she had sex with her Alsatian. She went into anaphylactic shock from the dog's sperm. I do not condone sex with animals, but it does happen out there in the real world, and I just wanted to point out that there are very real risks.

I have learnt a lot about sexuality from knowing articulate women, who have taught me about what it feels like to be a woman: to have a clitoris rubbed, to be penetrated, all in words that I can relate to as a man. I have learnt about aspects of the

G-spot and 'phantom orgasms', where the uterus contracts after a woman has had a hysterectomy.

Although I am an expert in the area of women's sexuality, if I was being intimate with a woman and she faked an orgasm I still wouldn't have a clue. You can't fake a wet vagina but you can fake an orgasm. One of my lesbian colleagues in the US told me that she and her partners prefer gay male to gay female porn because they feel it is more honest, since men can't fake an erection, and therefore my friends find it more authentically erotic.

I would like the experience of being a woman for about 20 minutes, during which time I would love to experience a multiple orgasm, foetal movements and childbirth, but then I would be happy to revert back to being a man!

Women's hormones ebb and flow over a month, while men's hormones are constant. Men do have a daily sexual peak, but it is at about 3 am when most people are asleep, hence the term 'morning glory' for a man's morning erection. Men need more direct physical external sexual stimulation as they get older, because by the time a man reaches his fifties and sixties his blood vessels may be silting up and since erection is a vascular phenomenon the nerves that control it can be affected as well. Alcohol and cigarettes are big factors in preventing men being able to get an erection.

Many men find it hard to understand the hormonal changes that women go through, such as premenstrual syndrome, as well as the other hormonal changes that take place at times of pregnancy and menopause. Often it's because no one has talked to men about this; their mothers would never have discussed the changes they were going through with their sons.

Andropause, the male menopause, is not as sharply defined and clear-cut as [is the menopause] in most women. For some women when they reach menopause they have one final period, while others may find that their periods dwindle or become heavier. But in men it is more diffuse as their testosterone levels alter in a variable fashion. Education is so important for men to understand any changes they are going through.

I had the usual sexually repressed childhood and used to get a perverse pleasure out of seeing how even any mention of sex would make my parents embarrassed. So I now believe that sex education is very important.

In 1976 the Education Department employed a colleague and myself to develop a sex education personal development course for teachers. We spent a lot of time on this programme, but when the teachers went back to their schools they found some of the principals very resistant to allocating time for the course. Those who did persist and teach the course found that as time went by the traditional expanding curriculum became more pressing, and the 'soft option' of personal development went by the wayside. This has been the same in university schools of medicine. I was instrumental in introducing sex education into the medical curricula, but gradually this has also been whittled away, with the excuse that there is not time to teach it with the pressure of the other coursework.

TIP: Having sex during pregnancy

It is fine to have sex during pregnancy as long as the woman is comfortable. It's important to have sex within the woman's comfort zone. As her stomach expands she may not like the traditional missionary experience, or to feel weight on top of her.

The position I recommend is for the woman to lie down over the edge or the end of the bed with her feet on the floor or supported so that her back is completely supported. Her partner kneels on the floor in front of her open legs, making him perfectly positioned to make love in a way that is comfortable for her. The other value of this position is that he is not bumping into her uterus, which will stretch its ligaments and hurt.

I do recommend to couples that they cease intercourse when the contractions reach every 10 minutes. After the baby has been born I always say a gentleman waits till I deliver the placenta. For some couples this is an extremely emotional and sexually charged time, and many couples can hardly wait to get home so they can make love. I remember a particular French couple, he told me afterwards he was so turned on he had an erection during the whole labour and birth.

Some men are reluctant to have sex during their partner's pregnancy because they believe they will harm the baby. On the other hand women often feel very sexual, especially if they are having a boy because of the extra testosterone in their body. I often have to convince the husbands that it is OK for them to have sex.

If women are worried about how they look I recommend intercourse from the rear, as no one looks pregnant from the back. It also means her belly can be supported by a duvet and bedding.

TIP: Expressing sexuality after an operation

It is important to help people find different lovemaking positions after an operation or injury. After having a mastectomy women often feel uncomfortable expressing their sexuality because they feel uncomfortable about their body. I suggest wearing a baby doll-style pyjama top to cover their breast and make them feel less self-conscious. When a woman has had a colostomy I encourage her to wear a sexy camisole.

I had a patient who had a hip that was fused and only had one leg that opened. There was only one position that she could make love in, and that was with one leg on the floor and lying face down, her body and other leg along the bed. She said that the problem with this was that she wanted to see her lover, so I suggested she use the sort of rear vision mirror used by cyclists or put a low mirror on the wall.

David Brown

David Brown and his wife Jane are the founders and principals of The School of ICASA Enhanced Sexuality, an independent training school for sexual and social skills in Bedfordshire, England.

In the 1980s he worked in the area of drug and alcohol counselling, which led to him working in the area of sexual dysfunction. In 1991 David and Jane were asked to help develop an impotence treatment clinic in Orlando, Florida. For the next two and a half years, they researched the subject of sexual dysfunction by studying the methods of Masters and Johnson, the Sex Therapy Institute of Boston and in particular the role of surrogate therapy.

In 1993 they set up their own school, ICASA (Inward Confidence and Sensual Awareness). Its training and techniques treat men and women with sexual dysfunction by using sexual surrogates. Their school is also affiliated with the Institute for Sex Education and Research founded by Dr Martin Cole.

David and Jane are also the Directors of Chelsea Medical Clinics Ltd, members of the International Professional Surrogates Association (IPSA) in the US and members of BEDS (British Erectile Dysfunction Society).

They contribute to Pulse Radio in Bradford, have appeared on television documentaries on sexual attitudes in Britain and have featured in numerous newspaper and magazine articles. David and Jane have been married for 27 years and have three children.

I was involved in counselling and rehabilitation work among drug addicts and alcoholics, and people with other life-controlling problems, back in the late seventies. I discovered that for addicts there often was a degree of sexual repression, misunderstanding, dysfunction and sometimes of course abuse, that lay behind the need to hurt themselves with substances.

In 1991 Jane and I were invited to help open a counselling side of an impotency clinic in the US, and I came to see how widespread and deep-seated sexual insecurity is. I valued the work that the doctors were doing in diagnosing physiological causes for sexual dysfunctions, and also the new treatments available. However, none of these things alone can fully take away feelings of inadequacy, humiliation and shame that deep-rooted sexual insecurity instils in a human being.

Seeing people become sexually liberated from negative feelings and realise their full potential is a privilege of my work. I have come to realise that helping people at this time in their lives is a gift. In that sense it has become my life's work. I didn't choose this work.

Sexual surrogacy is a therapeutic process that has been proven effective in treating psychogenic sexual problems that may otherwise remain untreatable. In men the most common complaints are fear of intimacy, premature ejaculation and performance anxiety. In women the most common are the inability to achieve orgasm, fear of intimacy, painful sex and rediscovering sexual confidence after menopause. Other conditions that affect both men and women are regaining sexual confidence following surgery, trauma or bereavement.

At The School of ICASA a potential candidate will first of all have a personal assessment consultation with either myself or Jane. Both of us are principals at the school. We will meet the candidate to determine what the presenting complaint is, take a case history, ascertain what the likely causes of the problem have been and determine whether ICASA Interactive Sexual Training would be an appropriate course of action.

If the candidate is a potential client he or she would then have a thorough medical examination. This will eliminate any physiological cause for the sexual dysfunction or, in other cases, will highlight a physical cause. It will also determine whether HIV or other STDs are present.

Following a medical report the potential client will then have an assessment with a clinical psychologist. This is to confirm the client's motivation and to protect any potential clients for whom sexual surrogacy therapy may prove too emotionally overwhelming. It will also identify any potential clients who may have fundamental psychological conflicts about sex or their sexuality. These conflicts would need some help to be resolved before a candidate would be deemed ready to embark on practical ICASA sexual training.

Following these mandatory protocols and assuming both the doctor and the clinical psychologist submit a positive report, which does not preclude surrogacy as an appropriate course of treatment, then the candidate may be accepted as a client of The School of ICASA.

Typically, a sexual training course consists of six two-hour sessions at The School of ICASA, which is situated in Bedfordshire, 40 minutes from central London, in a quiet country location.

Approximately half of every session is taken up with counselling, feedback and dialogue between the principals of the school and the client. The other half is in practical sessions, which include the sexual surrogate partner. The practical sessions allow the client to overcome the anxieties and resultant dysfunctions that they have experienced in intimate situations. The surrogate partner will enable them to practise their anxiety management techniques, sexual control techniques and other suggestions that will have been imparted to them during the first half of the session.

Each session is progressive. When a client has reached a point of new confidence and freedom from anxiety, he or she will progress to the next level of competence. Interactive Sexual Training of this kind enables the client to discover intimacy as a healing experience, free from the pressures, potential rejection and judgmental attitudes that the modern world has placed upon them.

At The School of ICASA the therapeutic relationship is a

three-way relationship involving the principal, the client themselves and the surrogate. Surrogate partners are very special people, defined by their ability to give of themselves emotionally and physically in order to help and unleash others.

Sexual surrogates are subject to regular medical checks. In addition, safe sex is part of my training programme, as is education on personal hygiene and respect for our own physical body and that of our partner. So long as adequate medical care is taken, and safe sex taught and practised, there is almost certainly far less risk of any STDs in the context of properly structured surrogate therapy than there is in many other sexual relationships.

It's very important to point out that the surrogate partner is not the client's counsellor. Our method ensures that the teacher or instructor, ie the principal, is the director of the programme. The client meets the surrogate partner only for the practical part of the session and even then the sessions are discreetly monitored by the director. Furthermore there is no contact between client and surrogate partner outside the therapy sessions – dialogue and feedback between sessions take place between client and director.

The client may be assigned more than one surrogate partner during the course of their programme and assigning partners is the responsibility of the directors. The client does not have the power of choice over this. Prior to commencing sexual training my clients will have been assessed by the clinical psychologist and emotional vulnerability will be one aspect that the clients are assessed for.

Our surrogate partners are trained to identify telltale signs of potential emotional connection during the practical sessions. The directors will also monitor the situation closely. From the very outset of a sexual training programme, it is emphasised very clearly that therapy is a means to an end and not an end in itself. The therapeutic experience is a transitory learning experience to enable the client to form relationships for themselves outside and beyond the therapy.

Clearly sexual surrogacy is not for everyone and for this reason candidate application procedures are very important.

The introduction of Viagra has made quite a few differences in the way that sexual dysfunctions are treated. Obviously impotence is no longer a taboo subject and men are much more able to talk to their GP about problems they may be experiencing. Viagra has, however, created a 'quick fix' solution for GPs and in that sense has let them off the hook from discussing the real issues and the real causes behind many sexual problems.

For the type of person who does not seek a quick fix, Viagra has made little difference, if any. Of course Viagra cannot meet the needs of somebody who is suffering from premature ejaculation, sexual aversion, fear of intimacy, performance anxiety, inhibited ejaculation or other such psychogenic sexual difficulty.

When it comes to education about sex and sexuality most of this is still very formal, very clinical and biological in content. Teaching about practical sexuality is still virtually non-existent in the UK. It seems to be assumed that because we are born as sexual beings that we know how to share that sexuality with other human beings instinctively. This is not true. Sexuality, which is not everything in a relationship but which is a major part of every relationship, is like an art form, which needs to be developed and honed until it is something that provides mutual fulfilment, pleasure and healing.

I believe that most people do not have expectations nearly high enough with regard to their sex life. There seems to be still so much emphasis on performance, objectives, goals, pressure, power, conception. All of these forces restrict people's expectations of their sex life, reducing it to something that we 'do' instead of it being a life-giving, healing and therapeutic experience that should be based on pleasure, mutual honour and respect. Moreover, most people, especially when they are young, only expect their sex life to remain active and pleasurable until they reach a certain age.

An expectation that we should be encouraging is for intimacy, and a right kind of sexuality, to be a fundamentally essential and active part of our life throughout our entire life. What's more, good and true sexuality within a relationship is free and yet many of the modern views regarding sexual issues seem to have somehow associated sex with power, money and wealth. So, yes, people's expectations about their sex life are probably pretty unrealistic because their expectations are not nearly big enough, not nearly high enough and not nearly long-lasting enough.

Exercise: Ten-tenning

This is a practical exercise that helps couples to communicate their most personal feelings in a non-threatening way. So long as fundamental love exists between them, this exercise is virtually certain to create changes and a deeper level of partner connection, creating an environment within which real change can be made.

The term 'ten-tenning' is used to describe this exercise, which is based on spending 10 minutes writing a letter to your partner – then exchanging the letter with your partner – and 10 minutes reading and responding to the letter written to you. This exercise may extend to 20:20, 30:30, 40:40 or even more depending on the importance and complexity of the subject about which you are writing.

When you are writing your letter to your partner, spend 10 undisturbed minutes writing it, expressing your innermost feelings about your sexual insecurities, anxieties, fears and aspirations. It is important that, as you write, you allow your true feelings to flow. Feelings must not be confused with beliefs. Beliefs are intellectual and objective; feelings are emotional and subjective. Your letter should express to your partner what you feel, what you have felt in the past and what you feel could happen in the future with regard to your sex life and your relationship as a consequence.

Your letter must never include any implied criticism or judgement of your partner. Your feelings are being expressed and they concern how you feel, what you are anxious about, what you fear and what you want for the future. This letter is not an opportunity to set any record straight or to effect changes in your partner by manipulation. It is a sharing of your heart with your partner.

If you don't have a current partner, complete this exercise and write the letter to an imaginary partner. Maybe, in order to help, you could think of a previous partner or a fantasy partner.

This exercise helps you to develop communication skills and openness that can be effective in helping to transform your partner's attitudes and behaviour, without hurting their feelings or causing any unnecessary conflict within your relationship.

Exercise: The power of your breath to reduce sexual anxiety

When you are anxious about sex, or fearful, nervous or even excited prior to sex, or even during sex, you are likely to breathe in a shallow or rapid manner, which will produce adrenalin in your body. The adrenalin reaction will then cause your muscles to become very tense and tight. Therefore it is vitally important that a man learns to control his anxiety and his adrenalin levels before and during sex by learning to breathe slowly and deeply.

This deep, slow breathing pattern will not only keep high levels of adrenalin at bay, but will also help to circulate sexual energy through the body and decentralise it from the penis during sexual activity, both in foreplay and during lovemaking. Practise becoming more conscious of your breathing and learn to breathe deeply, filling your lungs as though your lungs are a balloon that is filled with air each time you inhale. After filling the balloon to the fullest extent you must empty it completely with each slow, deliberate exhale.

For sexual control and anxiety management purposes learn to breathe in and out deeply and slowly through the nose.

Place one hand on your chest and one hand on your stomach, and take a deep breath. If you are breathing normally, your stomach hand will move, indicating that you are filling your lungs and they are pressing onto the diaphragm, which pushes the stomach out. If your chest hand moves instead of your stomach, then you are breathing in a hyperventilating manner.

Regularly take time to lie on a bed or couch. Monitor where you are breathing by placing one hand on your chest and one on your stomach. Breathe slowly and deeply in through your nose. Once your lungs are full, breathe slowly and deeply out through your nose. Once you have emptied your lungs, stop breathing for as long as comfortable (usually just a couple of seconds or so).

When you are uncomfortable, breathe in slowly and deeply again through your nose, then out through your nose, and then hold your breathing again for that short period. This exercise should be done regularly and intentionally until breathing deeper and slower becomes a natural thing to you. As a result, when you are in a situation that is going to raise your anxiety level (especially a sexual situation), concentrate on slowing your breathing down in order to help yourself relax.

The purpose of this exercise is to allow your body to get used to operating on less oxygen when you are resting, and to allow your body to adjust to lower levels of adrenalin.

Michael Castleman

Medical journalist Michael Castleman, MA, is the author of Sexual Solutions: For Men and the Women Who Love Them, *a classic self-help guide to men's common sexual problems that has been in print for 20 years and has sold 500,000 copies.*

Castleman answered sex questions for Playboy *magazine's Advisor column for five years between 1991 and 1996. His magazine articles dealing with sexuality have appeared in* Playboy, Self, Psychology

Today, Men's Fitness, Reader's Digest, New Woman *and* Cosmopolitan, *among others. In the late 1970s he worked as a family planning and sexuality counsellor at the Men's Reproductive Health Clinic, the first birth control clinic for men in the US.*

The Library Journal *called Castleman 'one of America's leading health writers' and in addition to* Sexual Solutions *he is the author of nine consumer health books, including* Blended Medicine, *a home medical guide that combines mainstream and alternative medicine for 100 common conditions;* There's Still a Person In There, *a guide to Alzheimer's disease; and* The Healing Herbs, *a scientific guide to traditional herbal medicine.*

His 10 books have a combined total of more than 2 million copies in print. His 1996 book on alternative therapies, Nature's Cures, *was nominated by the American Library Association as Health Book of the Year. That same year, he was nominated for a National Magazine Award for his coverage of breast cancer. Currently, Castleman devotes a good deal of his time to writing for sex and health-oriented Web sites, including a monthly Internet newsletter for Xandria.com, the sex toy company. In addition to Xandria.com you can read his work on PlanetRx.com, SelfCare.com, OnHealth.com, Depression.com and Alzheimers.com.*

He lives in San Francisco with his wife, a GP, and their two children.

Becoming a sex educator and writer came about by a rather strange accident. After college, in the mid-1970s, I worked as an administrator at a community health clinic in Ann Arbor, Michigan. We treated an enormous number of young people with sexually transmitted diseases, and did lots of contraceptive counselling and pregnancy testing.

Because so many of our clientele had sex-related issues, we decided to amass a patient-education library that dealt with STDs, contraception and sexuality. I was put in charge of assembling the library and in the process bought the two books by pioneering sex researchers William Masters and Virginia Johnson, *Human Sexuality* and *Human Sexual Inadequacy*.

This book contained the original M&J sex therapy techniques for dealing with rapid, uncontrolled ('premature') ejaculation in men. As it happened, I had that problem, and was quite bothered by it. I was fascinated to read how simple it was to cure. With the help of my girlfriend, now wife, I learnt ejaculatory control in about two weeks. I was elated. I suggested that we offer some sex counselling at the clinic. Ann Arbor is home to the University of Michigan and its medical school, which had (and still has) a noted sexuality programme.

So we brought in some experts who trained our staff in rudimentary sex counselling, and referred anyone with a more complex problem to the university. The programme was a big success.

Another of my jobs at the clinic was to write a biweekly health column for a local newspaper. I began writing about the sex counselling programme, and I've been writing about sexuality since then, for 25 years now.

My personal experience of having premature ejaculation bothered me a great deal, and helped me empathise with other people troubled by sexual difficulties. People with sex problems often feel desperate. Sex is so intimate and central to the human condition that when something goes wrong sexually, people often feel very unnerved. That's how I felt. I also felt elated when my problem got cured. For the several years I did clinical sex counselling, it was always a thrill to hear back from people whose problems were cured. Now I get thank-you notes about my writing.

I come from a sex-positive family. My parents, God bless them, began sex education for my brothers and me when we were very young, and sex was never a taboo subject in our home. So I didn't have the same struggles as many people from more repressed backgrounds. But I had been doing sex counselling and writing for a good five years before I got turned on to commercial sexual lubricants – and they were a revelation. My wife and I couldn't believe how much more comfortable and enjoyable they made sex. And we couldn't believe that we'd never known about them. Since then, I've become a major missionary for lubricants. I promote them whenever possible.

The myth is that 'normal' women self-lubricate adequately, and that only women with 'dryness' (menopausal gals and a few younger unfortunates) need commercial lubricants. Wrong, wrong, wrong. Plenty of women of all ages do not self-lubricate sufficiently to enjoy optimal pleasure from sex. I think everyone should use a lube every time. I do. But the studies show that few people do, only about one-third of Americans. That's why I've become a professional lube missionary. Someone has to spread the good word.

Sexual communication is, of course, a major issue in every relationship. Everyone talks about the need for sexual communication, but few experts help people get a handle on it. I've found that couple-oriented games can be a big help, especially the games produced by timefortwo.com and lovegames.com. My favourite timefortwo.com game is An Enchanting Evening. My favourite lovegames.com game is Speak Love, Make Love. Both of these games – and the others created by these companies – combine intimate communication with playful physical intimacy.

The hardest aspect of intimate communication is getting started. Games help break the ice and show people that they can discuss their love lives, the sexual moves they like and dislike, and do it in a loving, supportive way. Next, I think men need to make peace with their penises. This is a major, major issue for men.

My penis is just like yours – a little too small. Not that I think size matters all that much, you understand: my wife insists she loves the little guy just as he is. The sex books all say that my

3.75-inch flaccid member and 5.75-inch erection are smack in the middle of the average range. And the sex advice columnists all agree that men are too preoccupied with size anyway.

Preoccupied? Who, me? Well, maybe yours truly would be less preoccupied if all the so-called experts out there stopped pontificating that 'size doesn't matter', when every red-blooded man knows that it does. Maybe I'd be less preoccupied if the experts came out with the straight dope on what we average Joes – or should I say, Dicks – can do to help our tube steaks look their best... short of self-mutilation.

But no, nobody has ever done that. So I had to do it myself. Along the way, I discovered that there's a great deal more to penis size than the sex books and advice columnists explain. I also reaped an unexpected dividend: I made peace with my penis. You can, too.

'Men are obsessed with penis size,' says Palo Alto, California, sex therapist Marty Klein, Ph.D. 'During more than 20 years as a sex therapist, male clients have raised the issue so many times, I've lost count.'

Some years ago, for a magazine survey, 1,000 men were asked how they felt about the size of their penises. Almost every respondent said he was too small and wished he were larger. How many guys are significantly smaller than average? Not many. 'I'd estimate 5 per cent,' says Baltimore urologist James Smolev, MD, an assistant professor of urology at Johns Hopkins, who has seen thousands of penises up close during more than 25 years of practice. How many are larger? 'Maybe 10 per cent,' Dr Smolev says.

And how many are truly huge? 'Very, very few,' says noted New York City sex educator Betty Dodson, Ph.D., who organised group sex parties in the 1960s and 1970s, and saw (and did several other things with) thousands of penises. 'The vast majority were average, or a little bigger or smaller. I recall only a few guys I'd call really enormous.'

So where do average-size men get the idea they're too small? 'From pornography,' explains Richard Pacheco, a male porn star of the 1970s, now retired. 'The men in porn are a self-selecting group. Only the guys with the biggest dicks audition.'

The only penises heterosexual men get to see really up close – other than their own – are the ones in X-rated media. The men in porn are selected for their enormous endowments. They REALLY ARE significantly bigger than the vast majority of the rest of us. Porn penises are the standard against which men judge themselves, and that standard is seriously skewed towards Goliaths.

As a result, all of us Davids of the world are justified in believing that we have one of the smallest penises we've ever seen. In addition, men look down on their own penises from above, which makes them look even smaller, Pacheco explains. But they view porn penises from other angles: 'So many of the penis shots are photographed up from underneath. That makes any dick look big.'

For the record, the average flaccid penis measures 3 to 4 inches in length, but this is a rather 'soft' figure, as it were, because it depends on several factors. Most men notice that the size and hang of their penises vary. Sometimes they're shrivelled and weird looking, other times larger and nicely hung. More on this later. Flaccid size also depends on how much you stretch your organ while measuring it (most men pull hard) and where you measure from – the top of the penis to the base, where it attaches to the lower abdomen. As for the erections, the typical hard-on measures somewhere in the range of 5 to 7 inches, with the same caveats.

Flaccid size has nothing to do with erection size, says Martin J. Resnick, Professor and Chair of the Urology Department at Case Western Reserve University in Cleveland. It's quite possible to have a flaccid penis on the small side, but a 7-inch erection. In general, the smaller the flaccid penis, the more length and girth it gains in erection.

Whether flaccid or erect, penis size depends on the amount of blood that enters the organ through the pudendal arteries, and the amount contained in the penis's central corpus cavernosa, the spongy tissues that become blood-engorged during erection. Many things can affect penile blood supply:

- *Diet.* No doubt you're familiar with exhortations to eat a low-fat diet to prevent heart disease. Maybe more men would heed this advice if the American Heart Association added that a low-fat diet also helps penis size. A diet high in fat, particularly animal (saturated) fat, raises cholesterol, which narrows the arteries, including the ones that carry blood into the penis. High cholesterol increases risk of erection impairment, according to a study by Ming Wei, MD, of the University of South Carolina Medical School. Tests of 3,250 healthy (non-diabetic) men aged 25 to 83 showed that compared with those whose total cholesterol was below 240 mg/dl, those above 240 had twice the risk of erection impairment from poor blood flow. (A high-fat diet also increases the risk of prostate cancer.)
- *Smoking.* As if you need another reason to quit, smoking accelerates arterial narrowing, which is why smokers are at high risk for heart disease. Cigarettes hit men below the belt as well.
- *Relaxation.* The pudendal arteries are surrounded by smooth muscle tissue. When men feel anxious, explains sex therapist Dennis Sugrue, Ph.D., of Bloomfield Hills, Michigan, President of the American Association of Sex Educators, Counselors, and Therapists (AASECT), this muscle tissue constricts, limiting blood flow into the penis. But as men relax, this muscle tissue also relaxes, allowing increased inflow. (Viagra produces erections by relaxing this muscle tissue.) In addition, anxiety triggers the 'fight or flight' reaction. This reflex sends blood away from the central body,

including the penis, and out towards the limbs for escape or self-defence. But as men relax, more blood becomes available to the penis. 'When men become distressed about their size,' Dr Klein says, 'the anxiety may, in fact, contribute to penis shrinkage. If you want to be all you can be, relax, and stop worrying about it.'

- *Warmth.* You've probably noticed that in draughty, chilly changing rooms, your penis seems to shrink and your scrotum hugs your body tightly. But after a hot shower, your penis looks larger and your scrotum hangs much lower. Warmth is relaxing, Dr Resnick explains, which increases overall blood flow into the penis and encourages the scrotum to hang lower.
- *A comfortable, committed relationship.* Sure, one-night stands are fun and new relationships can be exciting, says Louanne Cole Weston, Ph.D., a sex therapist in Fair Oaks, California. But they also involve intimacy with women you don't know very well, if at all. That can produce anxiety. A familiar lover may not be as exciting as a new one, but familiarity allows you and your penis to relax, which helps your member look its biggest and best.

In addition to increasing blood flow into the penis, here are two other size-enhancing suggestions:

- *Lose weight.* 'When a man has a big gut,' Dr Sugrue explains, 'excess fat tissue surrounds the base of his penis, and his penis looks smaller. In [American] football, the backs, who tend to be trim, often kid the linemen, who are fatter, about their penis size. The backs get away with it because they can run faster.'
- *Exercise.* Working out helps control weight. In addition to regular physical activity Dr Smolev recommends abdominal exercises to reduce any fat pad above the base of the penis.

> But exercising the penis doesn't help. The sex media sometimes refer to the penis as the 'love muscle', which implies that, like the biceps, certain exercises may buff it up. 'The penis contains smooth muscle tissue,' Dr Klein explains, 'but that's not the kind that gets bigger with exercise.'

If you enjoy playing with sex toys, two devices may temporarily boost your erection size – cock rings and vacuum constricting devices, generally known as penis pumps.

Cock rings

Cock rings are rubber or leather doughnut-shaped devices that tightly encircle the erect penis. Typically used to help maintain erection, they may also provide a little size boost – just don't expect miracles.

Blood circulates in and out of the penis both when it's flaccid and when it's erect. The arteries that carry blood into the penis run through the centre of the organ, so during erection, as blood fills the penis's spongy erectile tissues, a cock ring doesn't keep blood out. However, one of the two veins that carries blood out of the penis, the superficial dorsal vein, runs close to the organ's outer skin (on top).

As the penis expands in erection, both the superficial and deep penile veins naturally get somewhat compressed, which restricts blood outflow and contributes to erection. A cock ring restricts outflow a bit more by compressing this superficial vein. The net effect is somewhat greater blood build-up in the penis, and a slightly larger, firmer erection. On the other hand, cock rings may constrict the urethra, Dr Smolev says, and interfere with ejaculation.

There are two kinds of cock rings – adjustable and nonadjustable. If you're at all concerned about damaging your penis (bruising is possible from a ring that's too tight) use an adjustable ring. 'Some guys swear by cock rings,' Dodson says. 'Others say they do nothing.' Try one and see for yourself.

Penis pumps

Penis pumps create a partial vacuum that draws blood into the organ, resulting in temporary size enhancement. They are usually used to produce erections in men who otherwise can't raise them. Once an erection has risen, pump users roll on a constriction band similar to a cock ring to help maintain turgidity. 'Vacuum devices are excellent, reliable, safe and effective,' Dr Smolev explains, 'but they're also cumbersome.'

Even if your little guy has no trouble rising to attention, pumps can be used for temporary size enhancement. Models differ, but all include a plastic tube that fits over the penis, fitted with a pump operated by using a hand bulb. You squeeze the bulb, which evacuates the air from the plastic tube, drawing blood into the penis. Just remember, the effect is temporary.

Surgery

You might have seen ads that run along the lines of 'Give Yourself a Major Confidence Boost: Penis Lengthening and Enlargement', with the phone number of a urologist. Surgical enlargement might boost your self-esteem. Then again, it might also destroy it.

Two surgical approaches are available. The more popular is penis lengthening. It's based on the fact that you have more penis than what hangs between your legs – the penis also extends into your lower abdomen. The internal penis is held in there by the penile suspensatory ligament. Cut this ligament, and much of the internal penis emerges from the lower abdomen, adding about an inch to the external penis.

But this procedure also has a significant down side, according to Dr Resnick. The suspensatory ligament is what makes an erection stand up. A surgically lengthened penis still gets hard normally, but it no longer salutes. Instead, it hangs down between your legs, requiring you or your lover to direct it by hand into erotic openings.

The other surgical option is girth enhancement. This is a two-step procedure involving fat removal (liposuction) from the buttocks, then reinjection of that fat under the penile skin. The before and after pictures offered by urologists who perform this procedure show pencils transformed into bratwurst. But again, there are down sides. The fat injections may not 'take', and if they take unevenly, you may wind up with a lumpy, mutant-looking dick.

Many experts in this area advised against surgical enlargement. Dr Resnick said it's 'not recommended. Infection and deformity are possible'. Dr Smolev was even more emphatic: 'Any operation to lengthen or thicken the penis should be outlawed.'

'You couldn't pay me to have my penis surgically altered,' Dr Klein says. 'The stories I've heard are horrendous.' There is, however, one type of minor surgery that's safe and can make the penis look larger, Dr Smolev explains – 'Liposuction of the suprapubic area.' That's the fat pad in the lower abdomen above the penis. 'If you eliminate suprapubic fat, the penis looks bigger.'

Most men may want larger penises, but ironically, the tiny group with large penises generally don't consider their humungous endowments a cause for celebration. 'This may come as a shock to men,' says southern California sex therapist Patti Britton, Ph.D., President of the Foundation for the Scientific Study of Sexuality, 'but many women are afraid of big penises. A large penis can bang into the cervix during intercourse and hurt the woman.'

'Back when I was involved in sex parties,' Dr Dodson recalls, 'every now and then we'd get a man with a really big dick. People would ooh and aah, but most of the women wouldn't go near them. They said, "No way you're putting that thing in me." Most wouldn't even take them in their mouths. I talked with a few of these guys, and they all said that having a huge cock was more of a burden than a joy.'

Even in pornography, enormous assets are not always, well, an asset. Richard Pacheco was one of the few X-men with an average endowment. 'I used to joke with my wife that I had the smallest cock to ever hit the big time.' He auditioned despite his size, or lack of it: 'I went in naive. At my first audition, I thought acting counted. Next thing I knew, I was a porn star, and the audience assumed I had this huge cock simply because I was in porn. But everyone in the industry knew I was on the small side.'

Ironically, Pacheco's average-size cock helped keep him in porn work: 'A lot of the women used to request me for anal scenes. Because I was smaller, anal sex with me was more comfortable for them.'

'Women are right,' Dr Klein says. 'Men are too preoccupied with their penises. Some women may be into size, but I've counselled thousands of couples, and I can't recall any women ever raising it as an issue. Men hung up on penis size don't understand good sex. Penis play can give a man great pleasure, but the best way to impress women with your prowess as a lover is to find creative ways to give them pleasure without using your penis. Use your tongue instead.'

'I've had hundreds of cocks inside me,' says Dr Dodson, now 71 and still doing it. 'There's nothing worse than a big dick on a guy who doesn't know how to use it. It's a nightmare. He plunges in before I'm ready. He bangs into my cervix. It hurts. I'd rather fuck a guy on the small side who knows how to use his tongue on my clitoris than a guy with a big dick who thinks that stuffing that turkey inside me is all there is to sex.'

In the old blues song, 'It Ain't the Meat, It's the Motion', a woman sings: 'It ain't the meat, it's the motion/That makes your momma wanna rock/It ain't the meat, it's the motion/It's the movement that gives it the sock.' Although Dr Dodson prefers a tongue on her clit to a penis in her vagina, she agrees with the song. 'To men, sex means fucking, which is fine as long as they know how to use it. Every man thinks he's a champion cocksman, but believe me, not many are. The marks of a good cocksman are his patience, gentleness and sense of rhythm.'

Here are Dodson's suggestions for skilful use of what's between your legs:

- *Don't plunge in the moment a woman spreads her legs.* Go slow. Give her time to get hot. 'It takes my pussy 15 to 20 minutes to relax and open up enough to accept a cock comfortably.'
- *Use a commercial sexual lubricant.* 'Use lube on both her pussy and your cock. Lube makes entry so much more comfortable.'
- *Don't push in deep right away.* 'The most sensitive parts of the vagina are the lips. Use your cockhead to tease her lips. Then run it up to her clit. And even after you've gone deep, pull back out and tease her vaginal lips with your cock.'
- *Enter slowly.* 'I've always preferred to be on top. That way I can control the speed and depth of entry. In my experience, most women share that preference. And if the man places his fist on his lower abdomen, the woman can rub her clit against it, which is very enjoyable.'
- *Cultivate a rhythm.* 'Don't just pump in and out furiously. Go for a slow, sensual rhythm – in, out and around with an awareness of how the woman is moving.'
- *It ain't the meat, it's the clitoris.* 'I wish men would get over their preoccupation with penis size. If you want to please a woman, focus on her clit. Fondle it gently, and especially lick it. That's much more enjoyable than feeling impaled on a cock of any size.'

But with all due respect to the clitoris, many women enjoy the feeling of having a penis deeply filling their vagina. 'Some women love deep penetration because it makes them feel closer to the man,' Dr Britton says, 'with a more intimate connection to him. And men like it because it makes them feel larger.' The good news is that deep penetration depends less on penis size than on sexual position. (On the other hand, for the few men with unusually large penises, deep penetration should be avoided because of the possibility of hurting the woman.)

Britton was a consultant in the creation of the instructional video, *The Complete Guide to Sexual Positions*, in which couples enthusiastically demonstrate 100 different ways to get it on. The narration points out which positions allow especially deep penetration. Here are a few to try:

- *Man on top.* The standard missionary position doesn't allow particularly deep penetration, but a few variations do. With a pillow under the woman's hips to raise her a bit, she bends her knees over her chest, then you kneel between her legs and enter her. Or hold her legs straight up over her head.
- *Woman on top.* This position allows the woman maximum freedom of movement. Encourage her to experiment with variations that give her a filled-up feeling.
- *From behind (doggie style).* This position allows some of the deepest penetration. In this position, even an average-size penis can bang into the cervix and hurt the woman. Enter slowly and be careful not to thrust too deeply. For an erotic variation, try this one with the woman standing and bent over the back of a sofa with you behind her.

'It's such a shame that so many men feel sexually inadequate because of their penis size,' Dr Dodson says. 'I should mention one other aspect of being a good cocksman. Enjoy your dick. It's fine as it is. Make peace with it. You'll be happier – and you'll have better sex.'

Then I think men need to make love the way women generally prefer. It makes women happy, and it prevents, and cures, many of men's sex problems. This was the message of my book, *Sexual Solutions: For Men and the Women Who Love Them*, which has not been out of print in the US for 20 years. Women's preferred love style involves leisurely, playful, whole-body sensuality that includes the genitals but is not fixated on them.

The whole body is a sensual playground. Women often complain that men explore only a few corners of it – and do that roughly and non-sensually. Men often complain that women want 'too much' whole-body foreplay. The fact is, men need an equal amount of it in order for their penises to work right.

All-genital sex, the kind depicted in pornography and written about in the men's sex magazines, is what men grow up thinking is the way to do it. *Au contraire*. Ask sex therapists and they'll all agree that genital fixation is a prime cause of both premature ejaculation and many of men's erection problems. (It's why so many male porn stars have such trouble getting it up and keeping it up.)

The body, male and female, needs whole-body, non-genital love play to relax and become fully aroused. The love style most women prefer is the same programme sex therapists recommend to prevent and cure premature ejaculation, and to deal with many erection problems – de-emphasising the penis and focusing on whole-body sensuality. Hence my message to men: make love the way women say they prefer. The woman in your life will be happier. And you'll have fewer sex problems.

> **TIP: How to improve your love life**
>
> Any regular moderate exercise helps one's love life. Regular moderate exercise (brisk walking, swimming, biking, yoga, dancing, etc) enhances awareness and enjoyment of the body. That's good for sex. Any regular moderate exercise helps improve self-esteem. That's good for sex. Any regular moderate exercise has mood-elevating, antidepressant value. That's good for sex. Any regular moderate exercise helps with weight control, which, in most people's view, enhances their attractiveness to sexual partners. That's good for sex. Any regular moderate exercise helps improve overall physical vitality. That's good for sex.

Bill O'Hanlon

Bill O'Hanlon, MS, was born in Omaha, Nebraska. He has been a therapist since 1974. He has authored or co-authored 19 books and has published 39 articles or book chapters. His most recent books are Try and Make Me! *and* Collaborative, Competency-based Counselling and Psychotherapy: A Basic Manual for Interviewing, Intervention and Change.

His books have been translated into French, Spanish, Portuguese, Swedish, Finnish, German, Chinese, Bulgarian, Turkish and Japanese. He has appeared on Oprah *(with his book* Do One Thing Different*),* The Today Show *and a variety of other television and radio programmes. Since 1977, Bill has taught over 900 therapy seminars around the world.*

Bill has been a top-rated presenter at many national conferences. He is a licenced mental health professional, certified professional counsellor and a licenced marriage and family therapist. His passions are playing guitar and writing songs, reading, watching films, teaching seminars and sex. He is married and has three grown-up stepchildren and one biological child. He lives in New Mexico, US.

My journey to help people has been a strong force in my life. When I was younger I was very depressed and came to the point of suicide. A friend convinced me to stay alive, but after I agreed to stay alive, I was faced with the dilemma of finding out how to be less miserable. As a result, I became obsessed with learning how people decreased their unhappiness and found ways to be happy in life. This quest eventually led me to psychotherapy.

My standards were very strict, though, when it came to approaches to therapy and change. I was only really interested in methods and philosophies of change that were effective (and later I added the criterion of respectful, as I came across so many approaches that seemed to me disrespectful of people who were suffering). The approaches that seemed right to me were very practical and aimed at helping people change, not just get insight into why they had problems. I became very fascinated with methods of brief therapy; helping people change rapidly and get on with their lives. Most therapy in those days (late 1970s) was long term, so I was going against the trend.

I had a professor in both undergraduate and graduate university studies who specialised in sexuality and opened that area up very compellingly for me. One of the things that drew me to sex therapy was that it was usually brief. Another is that I was raised Catholic, with a fair amount of shame about what was happening 'down there', as the priests would refer to our sexuality. I also was trained in marriage and family therapy and began to do a lot of couples therapy, which naturally included lots of sexuality issues.

I learnt that most people are very ashamed of their sexuality or their bodies in some way and that helped diminish my own body and sexuality shame. I am interested not just in helping people understand why they developed problems, but in helping them change in the directions that they desire. In this, I was greatly influenced by one of my teachers, Milton

Erickson, an eccentric and creative psychiatrist/psychologist who lived from 1901 to 1980. I studied with him in the late 1970s and have considered him my mentor.

I began to divide the world of changework into two major categories:

1. Explanation/pathology-based therapies. Those therapies that are mainly focused on discovering what caused the problem (in the past, typically) and are mostly focused on what is going wrong. There are deficits and pathological processes within and around the person seeking help.
2. Change/solution-based therapies. Those therapies that are mainly interested in discovering what helps people change, mostly oriented to the present and the future. When they focus on the past, they seek to discover strengths, abilities, motivations for change and non-pathological aspects of the person seeking help.

Now, of course, these contrasts, like most distinctions, can be drawn a little too generally. However, this distinction has been helpful to articulate a change happening in therapy, and that I hope to further with my books and workshops. I became passionate about bringing about a change in the direction of the solution-based therapies, which has led me to teach over 900 workshops and write 19 books and 39 articles or book chapters. And I am really at heart a lazy guy!

There is more discussion about sexual abuse of women than men, but I think things are changing and we are coming more to equity in this area. I have been surprised my whole therapy career at how common reports of sexual abuse and molestation are. I was molested when I was younger (by my grandfather) and when I speak or write about that, people often commend me for being a man and speaking about it, so I guess the perception is that it is more rare for a man to speak up, especially in a public arena. When working with men and women in this area I don't work differently based on their gender. I individualise my work according to their issues, not their gender.

I have worked with boys with anti-social behaviour. It is important to focus on the behaviour and not see the child himself as having a so-called 'anti-social personality' or as being 'sociopathic'. These are behaviours that these boys do, and that leaves the problem more open to change than attributing it to a more fixed/set quality like personality.

One of the first things I do in therapy is to find some connection with such a boy. I have a friend who works in an adult male prison and he told me that he has to find something he likes, or loves, in his clients or he will not be effective with them.

The next thing I would be interested in discovering is if there have been times that the boy, or others who know can tell me, had the urge to do something anti-social or destructive and restrained himself. Often I find evidence of this early on and it gives me hope that the boy isn't totally without conscience, compassion or self-control.

If I can't get any connection to a troubled boy, or find an exception to his anti-social behaviour, I proceed by working with those around the boy, to create a context of consequences and accountability.

TIP: Steps to healing from childhood sexual abuse

1. Acknowledge to yourself (and to others if that is all right and important to you) what happened to you.
2. Take steps to ensure that you are not abused further by the person/people who abused you in childhood. This might involve criminal or other legal proceedings against them, not being alone with that person, or cutting off the relationship you had with them.

3. Get clear on what your abuser/s was/were accountable for (ie what they did to you) and what you were and are accountable for (your actions then and now). Challenge your own and others' attributions of blame or devaluing regarding the abuse, eg 'I must have deserved it', 'I must have brought it on myself', 'I liked the attention, so I let it happen, therefore I'm partially to blame', 'I am bad', 'You made me do it to you', 'You wanted it as much as I did', 'You're a slut'.
4. Make room for your feelings, perceptions and responses to the abuse then and now. Don't try to forget or get rid of your experience because it isn't normal, right or acceptable. Acknowledge and value all the aspects of yourself and your experience as an antidote to shame. This may involve publicly acknowledging the abuse or your experience. It may involve dialoguing with aspects of your experience from which you've been alienated.
5. Value your body. Stop doing things that injure or punish you physically or put you at risk of injury. Start doing things that value and enhance your physical wellbeing.
6. Change patterns of action, thinking and interaction that don't work. Find out what you've been repeating in those areas again and again that leads to pain, frustration or impasses. Make the smallest change that will make a difference and build on that change.
7. Challenge ideas about yourself and your life from yourself or others that blame you, invalidate or undercut your trust in yourself, or close down the possibilities for positive change.
8. No one has the 'right' answer for how you can heal and move on. Some people do it by remembering; some by forgetting. Some by forgiving; some by not forgiving. Trust your own sense of things and don't be dissuaded by books, television programmes, therapists or experts from what you sense is your path to healing.

8

Unchained Melody

The attitudes and values of family, society or carers impact enormously on the sexuality of people with disabilities. People who are intellectually, psychologically or physically disabled are frequently viewed as either sexless creatures or people whose sexuality is out of control. The idea that people living with disabilities have a right to a fulfilling sexual life is a relatively new concept, and one that is still problematic to many.

Often well-meaning carers, or the parents of people with disabilities (who are often their carers as well), are embarrassed when faced with the blatant sexuality of the person in their care. A particular sexual act, such as masturbation, is often viewed as 'troubling' or 'inappropriate', when the same sexual behaviour from a non-disabled person would be considered perfectly 'normal'.

There is still hesitancy in showing sexual videos, or providing sexual products, to people with disabilities. Often people caring for the disabled wait for a sexual issue to come up, and then discuss it individually, rather than assuming that the people in their care want to discuss sex broadly and in detail. While it is easier for people who are living independently to seek sexual information, finding appropriate products and services is another matter.

But for many people with disabilities the most difficult issue is getting in touch with their own sexuality. Many have a negative body image, and frequently feel that nobody will ever desire them, a view absorbed from the dominant culture's obsession with the perfect body being the way to sexual and emotional fulfilment.

Practicalities may make it difficult for some disabled people to stimulate themselves sexually: arm paralysis, shortened arms or limitations with their hands may make genital masturbation difficult. Visual impairment may make looking at erotic pictures or videos almost impossible.

The disability activists in this chapter have made their work challenging and overturning these soul-crushing stereotypes. They show that a lively erotic imagination is the key to sexual wholeness, and this has nothing to do with your level of physical ability or disability.

Challenging discrimination of another kind, against gay men, is the work of the final contributor to this chapter. In many Western countries progressive anti-discrimination legislation has meant that it is unlawful to treat gays differently because of their sexuality. However, despite legislative changes, discrimination against gay men, most notably by other men, continues to be widespread and pervasive. Almost any survey of young men (in particular) will show a virulent homophobia, which is puzzling and disturbing. As this is not unlawful, it is rarely challenged. The basis for this seems to be the classic fear of difference, but in the situation of sexuality-based hostility between men, it is punctuated by an almost hysterical fear of homosexual sex. In particular it is characterised by an obsession on the part of heterosexual men with anal sex. From male jokey asides about needing to 'keep your back against the wall' when a gay man is around, to verbal abuse like 'you take it up the arse, don't you?', many heterosexual men seem vastly more preoccupied than their gay counterparts with anal penetration.

If the results of this were not frequently so violent and damaging, this preoccupation would be sexually fascinating. When I worked on an online sex education phone service the section that received the most interest was the one on anal sex. It proved to be the area that had the most fear associated with it, with many men believing that if they enjoyed anal pleasure they must be secretly gay. This continues to be one of the most widely misunderstood areas of men's sexuality. Almost every female sex worker has had male clients who request to be anally penetrated – it seems to be one of the most frequently requested fantasies.

Our contributor works with uncovering the roots of homophobia in military men. The defence forces have in recent times gained an unpleasant reputation for being hostile and frequently dangerous places for openly gay men. Challenging and attempting to overturn this has been an extraordinary task.

Dominic Davies

Dominic Davies is a psychotherapist and clinical supervisor in private practice in London. He has over two decades' experience of working with sexual minority clients and is co-editor, with Charles Neal, of three volumes of Pink Therapy, *a guide for working with gay and lesbian issues. He is also co-author, with Tom Shakespeare and Kath Gillespie-Sells, of* The Sexual Politics of Disability: Untold Desires.

Dominic is a co-founder and active promoter of the Sex & Relationship Facilitation Project, an international project to promote sex and relationship self-empowerment for people with disabilities.

He lives in the East End of London with his partner, artist Lee Adams, and their three-legged cat.

Working with minorities has been such a passion in my life largely from self-interest. I am a member of two minority groups, being both gay and disabled. I have heard of and experienced discrimination and prejudice to 'my peoples'. I am also a member of a powerful, dominant group – men. This conjunction has imbued me with the belief in my worth as a human being and some confidence that I ought to have the same human rights as everyone else.

My passion for promoting good practice with both minority groups is a commitment to social justice, but again motivated out of self-interest! I like to feel I can make a difference to this world. Others have said that gay people occupy the role of spiritual conduits; they show a wider world another way of being a man or woman. We hold a mirror to straight society and say, 'What you hold so dear, maybe isn't the only way to be in this world.' This is perhaps reflected in how many gay people are involved in the 'helping professions': healthcare providers, educationalists and spiritual leaders.

I feel some kind of calling to assist society and the groups of which I am a member to get to know each other better, to learn from each other. I guess my writing has been motivated by a belief that I have something to say and want to say it. I have written widely on gay therapy issues and disability sexuality issues. I believe in sharing knowledge and helping people make use of theory and research. Much of my writing has been using other people's ideas and taking them to a wider or different audience.

My first *Pink Therapy* book, for example, was bringing the ideas of a lot of US-based therapists to a British audience. They were those that I felt had a cross-cultural relevance and which I had found useful as a therapist practising in the UK. By the third book, I think we're breaking new ground worldwide, and offering innovative British-based research and practice back to the world.

In my work, learning about how human sexuality can flourish in the direst of circumstances has been my biggest revelation – how creativity helps people find a way to access their sexual pleasure and drive. I am thinking specifically about disabled people's sexuality. Despite the odds stacked up against some people being able to participate in conventional sexual activities, they find a whole new way of making out. Like the dominance transfer experienced by many people with spinal cord injuries. The brain can't send arousal signals down to a guy's dick any more, and so with a bit of practice and some ingenuity it retunes an area of the body that can still feel sensation, ie above the break in the spinal cord. Hey presto – he can cum by having his earlobes stroked, or his neck caressed!

When we were doing the interviews for our book *The Sexual Politics of Disability* we heard so many stories of the creativity of disabled people in finding ways of having sex and enjoying themselves sexually. I guess that process, hearing those stories, helped my own confidence and sexual self-esteem. People with the most severe physical disabilities showed just how vibrant sexual creativity can be. After all, your biggest sex organ is not located between your legs but between your ears!

The most common assumptions that people have about sex and disability are that disabled people don't feel sexy and can't perform sexually. But there's also the opposite, that we are like some libidinous perverts salivating over the weirdest things. These are so clearly examples of scaremongering and scapegoating by the dominant group. Anyone who is prepared to get to know disabled people will know that we are just as sexual as everybody else. That means there are disabled people who have very low sex drives and rarely have sexual feelings, through to those of us who can't stop thinking about sex, and whose sexual frustration drives them through the wall.

In fact the lack of opportunity for safe, consenting sexual relationships is probably the biggest difficulty facing us. By not seeing us as sexual, and by creating myths to scare people away from sex with disabled people, we effectively deny them one of the basic human drives. Society has more or less accepted the need for disabled people to be fed, clean, accommodated and even to work. But society still has trouble with the idea of our need to be sexual, to parent, to have loving relationships. Sex is a basic human need and a basic human right. Yet there are many disabled people who never experience affirming, loving, sexy touch. Many disabled people die virgins. That's pretty heavy in the 21st century, isn't it?

I guess that gays, lesbians and disabled people are fighting for the right to love whom they choose and to be seen as of equal worth to the dominant 'norms' in society. Society creates myths and tries to scare people away from getting close to sexual minorities and people with disabilities. This 'creating of monsters' out of us serves to keep us in our place and to help able-bodied heterosexuals feel OK about themselves.

However, we know that 'normality' is a myth. People don't fit into nice neat either/or categories. Binary thinking dominates, but doesn't reflect the realities of human experience. For example, the average healthy guy about town could in an instant become a severely disabled, brain-damaged, physically restricted guy permanently destined to lie in a hospital bed, due to the chance hand of fate in a road traffic accident. This happens every day to hundreds of young men.

Almost everyone has a 'flaw' or impairment in their physical functioning at some point in their lives – something that makes them 'different' or 'not normal'. They may be overweight, wear glasses, lose their hair early, whatever. The myth of perfection and normality, the myth of the body beautiful denigrates and tyrannises all of us. We need to start widening our ideas about what constitutes beauty and sexiness. To practise extending our own personal boundaries of what and who we desire. To experiment with and question the narrow definitions and examples made available to us. To see the person inside.

Skin hunger and touch are perhaps similar issues for my gay male clients and people with disabilities, although both groups have different ways and opportunities of dealing with this. I know many gay men who go out cruising and have lots of casual sex as a way of trying to have their need for physical contact met. They may feel shame about their bodies and their sexual feelings and be alienated from their feelings. Disabled clients have a similar skin hunger and shame and alienation from their bodies, but probably have fewer opportunities for having sex. Some may get touched more often in functional ways – with bathing and dressing. But these kinds of touch probably don't satisfy the hunger for gentle, affirming touch.

I became involved in a recent photography exhibition (*Intimate Encounters* by Belinda Mason-Lovering) because I wanted to be part of the movement to create sexy images of disabled people. This will help integrate the sexual into the lives of people with disabilities, show us as sexy and being turned on, and challenge the notion of disabled people as asexual. It's an interesting project and perhaps only a small part of a broader picture, but one that I do believe breaks down stereotypes and challenges our preconceived notions about disabled people's sexuality.

In short I guess I'd like the general community to see sex minority people as different, but equal. There have always been people who are attracted to the same sex, in all cultures and throughout time. Sometimes we're held in high status, at other times we're imprisoned and killed. I'd invite people to reflect on just what is so threatening about same-sex attraction.

TIP: Get to know your body

My main tip, for both sexual minorities and for disabled people, is: get to know your body. Many of us have grown up with messages that our bodies aren't to be trusted, that there is something depraved or wrong with getting aroused by the same sex. It can lead us to become quite shut off sexually. All the attention goes into quick, genital sex and this can then become dull, so we keep the variety up by changing partners! This is fine, but there is a whole lot more we can be doing. This is a basic sex therapy technique and works pretty well for most of us, whether we have sexual problems or not. It takes the pressure off performance and puts it back into pleasure.

Find a partner who will tease you with their touch, to caress parts of you that aren't normally touched in sex. I suggest you force yourselves to stay away from genitals for the first couple of times you practise this and to have a massage, experiment with different types of pressure, different fabrics caressing your skin, different smells (leather, silk, cotton, essential oils in massage, etc). Take turns in pleasuring each other in this way and, very important, give your partner feedback about what's great and how it could be improved. Enjoy!

George Taleporos

George Taleporos is a 25-year-old consultant, activist and academic from Melbourne, Australia. His parents are Greek immigrants who arrived in Australia as teenagers. At 18 months of age George was diagnosed with Spinal Muscular Atrophy, a neuromuscular condition that causes severe muscle weakness. He was sent to a school for children with severe disabilities and throughout his primary years was occasionally integrated into a mainstream school. It was not until high school that George attended a mainstream school full time.

Today, George has completed a Bachelor of Arts with first-class honours at Monash University, specialising in psychology, sociology and business disciplines. He also holds a Graduate Diploma in Educational Psychology and spent 18 months as a visiting academic at Monash University, teaching business communication. He is currently undertaking a Ph.D. in psychology at Deakin University, where he was awarded a postgraduate scholarship. George also conducts training and consultancy work in the disability field and teaches psychology at Deakin University.

George uses a motorised wheelchair for mobility and a machine during the night to keep him breathing. He relies on his parents and personal attendants for assistance with daily tasks. He describes himself as a disability activist with a slant towards the sexuality and interpersonal relationship issues that affect people with physical disabilities. George is also an experienced speaker, having addressed various AGMs, conferences, launches and forums, including keynote addresses at the NSW Post School Options state conference and the Pathways 2000 national conference in Canberra. George was a key player in establishing the Accsex network, a lobby group that addresses issues of access to sexuality and human relationships for people with disabilities. Individuals can subscribe to this group's e-mail list by sending a blank e-mail to ACCSEX-subscribe@yahoogroups.com.

I have always been fascinated by sex, sexuality and interpersonal attraction. In my late teens, I spent a lot of my time either thinking about sex or talking about sex. I guess that is not unusual for a teenage guy. But for me it became problematised, because I am a person with a physical disability. Unlike able-bodied people, I didn't have access to sexual affirmation, and my opportunities for sexual exploration and release were severely limited by my disability and by society's negative attitudes towards physical difference.

I began to wonder about the sexualities and sexual experiences of other people with severe physical disabilities like my own. When I completed my undergraduate degree in social science, I sought out opportunities to further my credentials, while simultaneously learning about the interplay between sexuality, body image and physical disability. This is now the topic of my current doctoral thesis in psychology at Deakin University, Victoria.

My research is aimed towards learning about the feelings and experiences of people with physical disabilities about sexuality and body image. It utilises both qualitative and quantitative techniques, ie focus groups and a survey. The focus groups told me a lot about the kinds of difficulties and barriers to sexual expression that are associated with having a physical impairment.

Meeting potential partners is a major problem for people with a disability and participants commonly spoke of their experiences of rejection and their frustrations with being single. As we expected, we saw that people with less severe disabilities experience fewer barriers, and people with more profound disabilities the greatest number. However, all people with disabilities find ways of adjusting to their physical difference. Positive feedback from significant others was discussed as greatly assisting the person with a disability to build a positive self-image, and to feel good about their body and their sexuality.

The survey data, which is yet to be analysed, will assist us in building a psychometric test of disability-specific sexual and body esteem. It will give us an idea of the differences that exist between people with and without disabilities in the area of sexuality and body image. It will also inform us about how these variables impact on aspects of psychological adjustment such as depression, stress, anxiety and self-esteem.

The English academic, Tom Shakespeare, inspires me. He is a co-author of a fantastic book called *The Sexual Politics of Disability*. I read this book while I was in my honours year and it really struck a chord with me, because he said many things that I felt were true about sexuality and disability. The book confirmed what I believed, and still do, that the difficulties that people with disabilities face in the area of sexuality are largely caused by social forces.

An organisation that has done something about this is The Outsiders, an English club based in London, which was set up to help people with disabilities find sexual partners. It operates the annual Sex Maniacs Ball, which brings sex activists from across Europe together for a night of fun and debauchery. I really support it and think that any effort to get marginalised people together is a good thing. There's a great deal of strength that comes from belonging somewhere and being accepted as the person you are – it appears to me that this is what a group like The Outsiders can do. I commend the organiser, Tuppy Owens, and everyone else who is making The Outsiders a safe and fun place for people to be. I hope that similar groups can spring up in other parts of the world, including Australia.

I believe that everyone has the right to experience sensual touch. For a variety of societal, physical and practical reasons, some people with disabilities have limited opportunities to experience this, and therefore they may seek out paid sexual services. It is important, however, that the provider of these services is not fearful of disability, and is sensitive to the specific requirements that the client may have. I recommend that the client is upfront about their disability when they make their enquiries. They may even try contacting their local sex worker organisation to find out which brothels are wheelchair accessible, or ask specifically to be put in touch with disability-friendly workers.

Before the Church took an interest in people with disabilities, many of us were simply left on the street to beg and die. In the Western world we have come a long way from this situation, to a point where it is now recognised that people with disabilities should be given the resources necessary so that we can live in the community. Institutions are generally not very good places to be, whether they are or are not run by a church. They are generally obsessed by rules and routine, there is commonly no privacy and no personal space and there is very little room for a person to express their sexuality.

In my 'research' I have seen a variety of sex toys but I'm yet to find one that works as well as a functional human hand. It appears to me that there are a lot more options for women in this area. If only occupational therapists would put a tenth of the time that they spend on splinting people's limbs into building a sex toy that will allow a guy to 'get off' I'll be a happier man.

Exercise: Planning for sexual time

When you have a disability, you may need to be more creative in order to express your sexuality. However, no impairment is exactly the same and people with different disabilities have different challenges. If you have an impairment that limits your genital sensation, spend some time exploring all the different parts of your body, especially your neck, your ears, your armpits and your nipples.

Close your eyes and focus on the sensation. If you have a partner, let them know the spots that feel good. Even though you may have lost the sensation in your genitals, this doesn't mean that they should be ignored altogether; you may simply need to become reacquainted with them.

Rub your genitals and enjoy the sensation on your fingers, stroke your genitals and your inner thighs and attend to how your body responds. Don't expect anything, just observe. Do these things in a sensual environment, depending on what turns you on.

If you have a disability, you may find that you have to be more proactive with your sexuality. You may have to 'plan' your sexual experiences. Don't let this put you off, because with planning comes anticipation and simply anticipating a sexy event can be pleasurable. For example, you may decide to plan an evening with an escort. Choosing an escort, or choosing the brothel you want to visit, can be a lot of fun. I think it is also very important to choose care workers who are accepting and affirming of your sexuality, because you may need them to facilitate your 'sexual lifestyle' in various ways. Try hard to avoid 'mothering' or 'controlling' carers. It is usually best to ask a few relevant questions in the interview stage to weed out those types.

Eugene Moore

Eugene Moore was born in the west Texas town of Odessa but at the age of one moved to southern California, just south of Los Angeles. After finishing high school, and in distress over his homosexual desires, he 'found Jesus' and ended up studying for the ministry at the Moody Bible Institute of Chicago, from where he graduated in 1975. Trying desperately to 'get over' his homosexuality, he went a step further and got married during his last year in Chicago. He and his wife then moved back to California, where he received a BA in Religious Studies from Vanguard University, a Christian liberal arts college. Having developed a passion for history, he then completed an MA in Social Sciences (history and anthropology) at the California State University, Fullerton. He began teaching in a large secular college and eventually became assistant professor of history at Vanguard University while completing another MA (social history) at the University of California, Irvine.

It was while teaching at Vanguard (then known as Southern California College) that his homosexuality finally burst out into the open, and in the span of literally a few minutes he lost his career and his marriage. He regards those days as the worst and the best of his life. With a mixture of devastation and elation he moved to the island of Rarotonga in the South Pacific to regroup and try to make sense out of what had happened. Building a house made of bamboo walls and coconut palm roof, he settled into a fairly idyllic lifestyle of spearfishing for his meals in the lagoon and socialising with friends who knew little of the homophobia that had driven him from himself and his home.

From there he moved to Hawaii, where he taught for the University of Hawaii community colleges and pastored the (gay-friendly) Metropolitan Community Church in Honolulu. Part of his university teaching responsibility included classes at Schofield Barracks for soldiers of the chemical warfare division. He never came out to them, or to any of his students, since the fear of homophobic reactions was still fresh.

After Hawaii, Eugene decided to make New Zealand his home, having visited there on several occasions. Enrolling for a Ph.D. in gay history at the University of Auckland, Eugene discovered a world of queer theory and a history that is largely hidden from view within academia, but that has such power to transform people's views when the veil is lifted. It was during this time that he decided to put his studies on hold and launched Full Spectrum Ltd, a consultancy specialising in creating inclusive environments for sexual minorities in large organisations.

He now specialises in military and law enforcement organisations, enjoying the challenge of working in what are regarded as the most homophobic professions in the world. He provides education throughout the New Zealand armed forces, police and customs service and the Australian armed forces.

In spite of prevailing opinion suggesting that attempts to change attitudes in military environments will be ineffective and resented, the work carried out by Full Spectrum is proving the opposite, with dramatic changes occurring among even severely homophobic individuals.

I have lived most of my adult life pretending to be heterosexual in every facet of life – family, work, religion, social, etc. I know the toll it takes and the essential inequities involved. And the tolls are not restricted to those of us who are sexual minorities – our heterosexual loved ones, friends, professional colleagues and the organisations in which we work also pay a heavy price when homophobia and the fear of homophobia are allowed to dictate the way people live and work.

However, the immediate reason that I got into this line of work was due to realising, during doctoral studies in gay history at the University of Auckland, that organisations needed help in understanding the issues for sexual minorities in the workplace, considering that New Zealand law forbids discrimination on the basis of sexual orientation. Most managers are thoroughly unaware of what the issues are and the steps needed to address those issues. Being aware of consultancies in the US that do this kind of work, I recognised a tremendous gap in New Zealand and Australia that was waiting to be filled in an area that many do not normally associate with sexual orientation issues – the workplace – and that by addressing those issues in a positive way that provides incentives for employers to create inclusive environments, the lives of gay, lesbian and bisexual people would be enhanced. People spend a tremendous amount of their lives working, and yet most gay people – even those who are out in the wider community – retreat into the closet at work. My original motivation was that the work needed to be done. My subsequent motivation comes from the fact that the work is much easier than I anticipated and the rewards are tremendous in terms of seeing organisations and lives improved.

After coming out of the closet and leaving the religious institutions that had played a central part in my life, I felt not only that my roots had been ripped out of the ground, but that I had wasted the best years of my life on an ideology that effectively made me hate who I really am, and that made the prospect of ever having a loving relationship with another human (towards whom I actually felt attracted) impossible. However, I now see that by studying and living among some of the most conservative elements of American Christianity, I can 'get through' to people for whom their religious beliefs are the foundation for their negative attitude towards homosexuality and homosexual people. By understanding their beliefs, worldview and consequent fears about homosexuality, I can demonstrate to them that I am not a complete 'other' who does not appreciate their position. And that makes them willing to listen to me. By understanding the arguments and biblical theology they use to defend their positions, I can answer those objections in a way that makes sense to them. But most importantly, I am able to demonstrate to them that they can retain their moral and religious beliefs about homosexuality being a 'sin', while at the same time treating homosexual people equitably and with respect, without feeling that they are 'promoting homosexuality'. Since the most ardent and organised opposition to the equality of homosexual people in Western society comes from what is commonly referred to as the 'religious right', having been a part of it for so long is invaluable in the work that I do.

Having done degrees in religious studies, cross-cultural ministries, social sciences (history and cultural anthropology) and social history, I've managed to develop an outlook on life that makes my practical work much more effective. For example, I am attracted to history primarily because of its ability to deconstruct the present. That is, history tells us the story of how we got to the present, the multitude of factors such as circumstances, ideologies, people and events that have constructed the world in which we now live and the 'reality' that people perceive. By going back over that story and analysing those factors, we are essentially deconstructing the present and looking at how all those factors contributed to a construction of the world as it is – including the perceived 'reality' of what same-sex attraction and relations are all about. And what I've found is that when you help people see the present as a product of all those factors, then they realise that the 'way things are' is not necessarily 'the way things should be'. Rather, it is just the 'way things happened to occur'. It destroys the omnipotence and omniscience of the present and reveals it to be the product of factors that could have created a very different 'reality' about homosexuality had those factors been a bit different than they were. I make the history of attitudes towards homosexuality (and a comparison of cultural attitudes) an integral part of my seminars because it transforms the way that people see the subject.

Similarly, my background in cultural anthropology has been invaluable in understanding the variety of attitudes towards same-sex desire and behaviour that occur within various cultures. Again, such an understanding serves to 'dethrone' our own peculiar cultural attitudes.

It is difficult to assess what the motives are for young men to commit violence towards men they perceive to be homosexual. I'm often not really sure of my own motives (which can be quite mixed) in any given situation – much less am I confident about assessing the motives of others! But overall, I'd say there are several possible motives that might drive young men to act violently towards gay men, and that those motivations may or may not be apparent to the perpetrators.

In some cases, it could be that the young man is acting out his own insecurities regarding his sexuality. This is not to say that the young man in question is necessarily gay, just that he may be experiencing some level of homosexual attraction, no matter how trivial. For male youth, who are raised to believe that to be considered heterosexual one must be 100 per cent heterosexual without a trace of same-sex desire or behaviour, even the smallest amount of the latter is enough to put some of them in a tailspin. There is no doubt that one of the 'strategies of denial', to use a term by Australian psychotherapist Vivian Cass, that is used by people who are desperately trying to deny their same-sex desires, is to lash out at homosexuality in others. Unfortunately this can take the form of verbal and physical violence.

However, one must be careful to avoid pinning all gay-hate violence on such people, as it effectively blames gay and bisexual men for their own persecution by making both the perpetrator and the victim 'homosexuals'.

Australian David Plummer, author of *One of the Boys: Masculinity, Homophobia and Modern Manhood*, has found that homophobic labelling begins very early for boys – primary school specifically – and reaches an apex in secondary school. This labelling is not restricted to boys who are actually homosexual, but can be attached to boys who are merely perceived as different: too smart, too well liked by teachers, not interested in sports, etc. Homophobia serves to define masculinity, and to effectively separate 'the men from the boys'. While many lessons can be gleaned from this, one is clear – that homophobia begins early and by secondary school it is a central part of male youth culture. It is hardly a wonder then that young men would be prone to lashing out at gay men.

Homophobia polices not only men's sexuality, but a dizzying array of non-sexual aspects of living – particularly in relation to male-to-male contact. Plummer speaks of a continuum of contact, with looking at each other on one end, moving on to a handshake, a pat on the back, a hug, a kiss and finally sexual intercourse. What determines whether any of these contacts are regarded as homosocial behaviour, which is acceptable, or homosexual behaviour, which is unacceptable, is homophobia.

What other logical reason is there that determines that up until the age of 10 or so, it is acceptable (homosocial) for males to walk with arms around each other's shoulders, and later that such behaviour is regarded as unacceptable (homosexual)? What is it that determines that in Eastern Europe it is acceptable (homosocial) for two males to greet with a kiss on the mouth, but in New Zealand such behaviour is regarded as unacceptable (homosexual), other than homophobia? Thus, homophobia and the fear of being homophobically labelled/persecuted by other males dictates to all males a vast array of rules governing their relationships with each other that effectively keeps them at an artificial distance from other males – and themselves. Homophobia and the males who enforce the fear of homophobia can even keep males from displaying normal human emotions such as crying. What other than homophobia keeps males from crying? What logic says that crying is a 'non-masculine' (and by implication, non-heterosexual) response to certain circumstances? Males hold back their tears because they don't want other males to label them as 'girl's blouses' or 'faggots'. Boys are thus effectively 'dehumanised' by homophobia and the fear of homophobic reactions from their peers.

When I first began working in military and law enforcement agencies, I anticipated difficult work! What I have found is that in what are widely regarded as the most homophobic professions in the world, amazing changes can take place when the right information is shared in the right way. I have personally witnessed men undergoing huge sea-changes in attitudes in as little as one hour. I could relate so many stories, including from men who admitted that prior to the awareness education they would have reacted violently to someone they knew to be gay. From new entrants to senior commanders, the story has been the same. In one particularly memorable briefing to top military commanders, an officer who had consistently expressed very strong reservations about even scheduling the briefing turned to the commanding officer and said that his mind had been changed. What had changed it, he said, was an understanding of what it would be like to live in the closet. He couldn't stand to live like that, and he didn't expect anyone else in his branch of the military to live like that either.

For him, it was an understanding of the damage done to individuals and by extension, to the organisation. For others, it can be very personal. One senior officer, after learning of the effects of parental homophobic messages and the effects of those messages on children who may have some degree of homosexual orientation, went through some significant rethinking about his attitudes and behaviours.

TIP: Coming out

Coming out to oneself is the most important step a person can take. Until one is willing to confront the reality of one's own sexuality, it is impossible to be honest with others. Coming out to others, on the other hand, is one of the most difficult things a person can do. It is fraught with danger and uncertainty, since one never knows how another person will react to the news. Many people choose to be very selective in the coming out process. And that is what it is – a process – not a once and for all event, since daily life presents innumerable opportunities to either tell the truth or avoid the truth.

I've been well and truly out of the closet for years, but it took years to become comfortable with it. However, I still fear disclosure in many circumstances. For example, I find it easy to be open about my sexuality while standing in front of a roomful of soldiers. But when I'm picked up from the airport by a military driver and in the car he asks, 'What are you coming to the base to do?', I feel quite anxious because I have no idea how he will respond to the news that he is sitting next to a homosexual man.

The more personal the relationship, the harder it is, I believe – because there is more at stake than with people who are at more of a distance. When I came out to my sister, to whom I am very close, it took me over two hours while sitting in her living room to get the words 'I'm gay' out of my mouth.

I suppose the only tip I'd give is this: that the closet is a demoralising, depressing, lonely, shameful and terrible place to live, and that coming out of it can be the most frightening, courageous and liberating experience(s) of one's life. Life outside the closet can be fraught with danger, but life inside the closet definitely is. The danger is to one's sense of self and wellbeing. Living courageously is infinitely better than living in shame – at least in my view. One thing is for sure – coming out will reveal who your real friends are! And it can be very surprising.

9

Celestial Spirit

The men in this chapter have been chosen because they have moved with the times, even challenging their own faith around issues of sexuality. Many religious beliefs underpin the structures of society, but are rarely examined. These men are trying to incorporate religion with sexuality in the Western world in which we live today.

Christian Church

The primary concern of the Christian Church is to defend and protect heterosexual marriage and the family, which it sees as the basis of Christian society. While there are some Christians, notably the Quakers, with a much more liberal view of homosexuality than the Catholic Church, all Christian teachings on sexuality follow from that principal concern of marriage and the heterosexual family unit.

Sexual intimacy with another person is part of the privilege of marriage, and so sex outside marriage, particularly with no intention of marrying or procreating, is seen as suspect and an indulgence of the senses. In extreme cases the Church has taught that this weakens the body and saps the moral courage of individuals. In an ideal Christian world, the faithful marry and stay married, and bisexuality and homosexuality are unknown.

Most of the Christian Churches have a clear opposition to homosexuality, and in the Catholic Church this comes right from the top, recently enshrined by a specific Vatican edict against same-sex relationships. The Christian Churches see themselves as shouldering no blame for preaching against homosexuals, claiming instead that the gay and lesbian communities are pushing a 'gay agenda' and 'encouraging' people to be homosexual, and that the Churches are merely responding to this.

Judaism

As in the Christian faith, Jewish people have wide-ranging views about what they believe to be sexually right and proper. Unlike other religions there is no official stance on many sexual topics. The concepts of sin, damnation and purgatory do not exist as in Christianity, hence the tortuous guilt is not experienced, but this is not to say that sexual repression does not exist.

The Jewish faith's reference to masturbation comes from the Torah, its holy books. In Genesis, Chapter 8, the 'spilling of his seed' is condemned, hence masturbation is not encouraged. At the same time human beings are seen as sexual creatures who express this in various ways.

Many liberal Jews argue that the teachings of the Torah were written thousands of years ago and that in the 21st century things are viewed differently. With regard to sex before marriage, sexual experimentation within a committed relationship is often considered acceptable, and homosexuality is not something that reflects sexual choice but is part of a person's being created in God's image.

Orthodox Jews believe that couples should not sleep in the same bed before, during and shortly after a woman is menstruating. This is interpreted as a way to increase passion in the relationship.

Buddhism

Although there are different schools, or traditions, of Buddhism, they are generally united in their view of the basics of Buddhist sexual conduct: to refrain from sexual misconduct. No particular sexual behaviour is forbidden per se, but they believe that we should be aware of the possible result of any sexual action in our lives. Buddhists are urged to refrain from behaviour, be it verbal or physical, which is likely to result in physical or mental harm, either to oneself or to others. You are responsible for your own actions, and the result of those actions.

Critics of Buddhism often claim that it doesn't have a strong moral code, which is not true, but it does not have a concept of sin in the Christian tradition. Instead it has the concept of karma (the cosmic law of cause and effect). Buddhism also urges that we follow the 'middle way', neither denying the body and its pleasures, nor becoming obsessed by them. The Dalai Lama spoke about the dangers of sexual preoccupation in the following way:

> Sexual desire, by definition, wants something, which is the satisfaction of desire by the possession of the other. To a large extent this is a mental projection, provoked by a certain emotion. We imagine the other in our possession. At the moment of desire everything seems agreeable and desirable. One sees no obstacle to it, no reason for restraint. The object desired seems to have no defects, to be worthy of all praise. But then everything changes with possession. Once the desire disappears – whether it considers itself satisfied, or time passes and weakens it – we no longer look at the other in the same way. The appearances of the once desirable object change and sometimes rapidly, suddenly. Some people admit they are stunned by this. The emotion they started out from is dissipated, giving way to a reciprocal misunderstanding. Each one discovers the true nature of the other, which up till then had been hidden by his or her desire. That is why there are so many broken marriages, quarrels, lawsuits and hatreds.
>
> (His Holiness the Dalai Lama, *The World of Tibetan Buddhism*)

Reverend Bill Huff Johnston

The Reverend Bill Huff Johnston was born in Sydney, Australia in 1939 and comes from a Presbyterian family. He trained in fine arts and became a potter, eventually teaching pottery in London, Cornwall and Devon. Creativity has always been his joy. In 1967 he moved back to Sydney and taught at East Sydney College. Four years later he moved to Canberra with his wife and three children. Since this time he has worked with the Institute of Arts at ANU University and been involved in the promotion of fine arts.

He has also worked with Lifeline, a charitable, non-denominational organisation, helping people with their problems. He has consistently supported women's liberation and the movement for gay and lesbian rights.

After lecturing in Canberra for 21 years, in his fifties he decided to do a theology degree. He has worked as a reverend since this time. He is one of the few ministers who counsels in the area of sexuality and is the official chaplain to the Eros Foundation, Australia's national political lobby group for the sex industry. He continues to work in fine arts, but also writes articles for the Eros Foundation's magazine.

I had always had a passion for helping people and was blessed with a loving family, good health and opportunities in life. I had worked on the night shift for many years with Lifeline, on their phone counselling service. I spoke to many people and helped with their issues of loneliness, guilt, anger, frustration, confusion and grief.

I felt that although I adore the potter's wheel I was driven by a need for something more. Artists, musicians, poets and dramatists think differently and have a different way of seeing life. Theology is also a different way of seeing life. I found it difficult at first, and while I was studying my teachers found me difficult, because my form of expression was challenging to them.

My background as an artist gave me the flexibility of seeing and expressing life from many different angles, therefore I challenged the ethics of the course I was studying. I finished my degree after studying New Testament Greek and Hebrew, as well as biblical, liturgical, historical and pastoral care used by hospital chaplains. When I finished my degree I felt that the spiritual side and the ethical side had come together for me in a creative way.

If I had done my theology course at an earlier age it would not have been as easy for me to be accepted by the Church. Anyone can study for a theology degree, but to be selected for ordination was very important to me. Historically clergy have been of three types: bishops, priests, who are in charge of a parish and deacons. Deacons traditionally are a position given to a new priest for a year. Going back to the New Testament there is another meaning, which is to go outside the parish totally.

My role now is involved with chaplaincy work, prisons, the university and counselling for people working in the adult industry. I am attracted to working with marginalised people, or people who don't speak the Church's language, rather than to be tied as a priest to just one parish.

I believe that sensuality and sexuality are the motivation for so much work that is visual, dramatic and creative. I see no shock value in nudity in painting, sculpture and photography, as the body can be given expression in any and every way.

I enjoy immensely the diversity of the work that I do. I feel I bring the expression of 'the Spirit in Life' to it. It is less definable and can be expressed in the spirit in dance and music, to make you feel better and motivate others and celebrate that life is good. When I am talking I am conscious of the visual, passionate joy in life. My whole role is to walk alongside people and be accessible.

If we have the chance to be intimate with ourselves, or with our lover, or God, or with people in our lives, and that takes the form of wonder, it's to be celebrated. I appreciate that life is the explicit part of sexuality, the implicit part of my faith and spirit.

I try to grasp a commonality with other human beings, be they university lecturers or sex workers.

> **TIP: Finding the joy in life**
>
> Many people don't give themselves the chance to rethink because it is too scary. There may be some people who will never give themselves the opportunity to expand in their life. This includes sexuality and spirituality. My way of finding joy is to start with the visual; the painter is able to see the beauty in everything. The beauty is in the eye of the beholder, be it a painting, pornography, or the opportunity to have an open mind to respond without prejudice. Give yourself time to re-evaluate your mindset.

Rabbi Shmuley Boteach

Born in 1966, Rabbi Shmuley Boteach is the founder and dean of the Oxford L'Chaim Society at the University of Oxford, where he served as Rabbi for 11 years. He has recently been appointed President of Michael Jackson's Heal the World Foundation, under whose auspices he co-founded the Heal the Kids Initiative. Author of 12 books, including the international blockbusters Kosher Sex *and* Dating Secrets of the Ten Commandments, *and the critically acclaimed* Moses of Oxford, *Rabbi Boteach's writings have featured in publications as diverse as* The Times *and* Playboy *magazine, which chose* Kosher Sex *as its main book selection for its 45th anniversary edition. His three books on relationships were each serialised over several days in the* Daily Mail *newspaper. His weekly essays have been distributed on the Internet for nearly a decade and have a vast following.*

He has appeared on all the major British, American, Canadian, Australian, Israeli and South African television and radio shows and was the subject of a major documentary in the BBC's Everyman *series.*

He has also been profiled in many publications, including The New York Times, The Washington Post, *the* Los Angeles Times, The Miami Herald, *the* New York Post, Time *and* Newsweek.

An internationally acclaimed speaker, Rabbi Boteach won the highly prestigious Times Preacher of the Year Competition in London just days before the millennium, and was also placed as first runner-up the previous year. In his winning address Rabbi Boteach won more points than any competitor in the competition's history.

Rabbi Boteach lives in New York with his Australian wife Debbie and their six children.

My journey to teach people about love and sex has been so important in my life because I am the child of divorce, and only now are we beginning to weigh the consequences of divorce on children. We became so blasé about divorce that we forgot how devastating it actually is for children. Divorce was such a common occurrence for children of the seventies that saying your parents got divorced was almost like saying that you had your tonsils removed, or that you fell over and scraped your knee when riding a bike. We now know that divorce scars children for life, and you never completely overcome it.

A man once asked me, 'Will getting divorced affect my children?'

I answered, 'What if you told them the sun wasn't rising tomorrow – would that affect them? What if you told them that their hope that everything works out in life would suddenly be snuffed out? That the two people who brought them into this world – the archetypal relationship that is responsible for their existence, has dissolved? After hearing this, they could only conclude, cynically, that life is accidental, that things don't work out, that the world is comprised of incongruent pieces of a puzzle that ultimately never fit.'

Hence, teaching people about love and sex has been a healing journey for me. I want to heal myself, and I feel that if

I explore and express my own belief in love, I will internalise the message and the scars will heal as best they can. (Although I have always maintained – perhaps cynically – that they will never heal completely.)

Sex is the ultimate expression of love, so the two subjects are not only interconnected but one is the outgrowth of the other. I know that today that is a very controversial statement, because we are a generation that prides ourselves on separating sex from love. Ideally I am one of those romantics who believes that they can't be separated, and that loveless sex is actually pretty bad sex, and is something that ultimately turns us off sex.

I also don't believe that we are the oversexed society that we think we are. I actually think that we are very undersexed, which is why we have to talk so much about it as opposed to doing it. Sex has lost its spark, it has lost its magic. If anyone asks what is the driving force of this day and age, it is not sex – it is money. This is the age of financial preoccupation.

There is not a plethora of sex channels on cable TV, but there is a plethora of cable channels such as CNBC, that provide 24-hour reporting on the stock market. Money is what we make love to today and our relationships with our partners and children have suffered as a result.

It is not true that Judaism has had a strict sexual code. On the contrary – that is one of the misconceptions about Judaism. Judaism always had an extremely liberal and life-affirming sexual philosophy. However, Judaism does teach that in order for eroticism to be preserved, there have to be certain borders and barriers that always have to be maintained, because total availability and accessibility in sex as well as in love would be the bane of marriage, and the destroyer of relationships. Hence Judaism instituted a period of sexual separation in marriage.

Women's sexuality has been transformed by the sexual revolution – to sum it up, female sexuality has become masculine. The mystery of sex has always been that women grounded men in more intimate and more emotional relationships. Men would never really have been involved in those relationships based on their nature alone, which is polygamous. But there was no one with whom they could share that lifestyle because women weren't game.

The sexual revolution in the 1960s did not affect men in the slightest. It was an entirely feminine revolution whereby women said, 'We can practise the same compartmentalisation as men', and they defined sexual maturity as that compartmentalisation. Women said, 'We no longer need love and sex coming side by side.' The result was destructive all round. One need only look at the numbers. Fifty per cent divorce rate. People marrying later than ever before. People don't believe in love, and 43 per cent of American women say that they no longer look to men as a source of their happiness.

Judaism has not been challenged by this, but nevertheless, it has a profound role to play in addressing this. On the contrary, who would have expected a book like *Kosher Sex* with its 'Stone Age' sexual ethics to have ever sold in large numbers to mainstream America?

First of all, all of us have a finite libido, and masturbation doesn't enhance that libido, certainly for men. It has been proven that sexual steam goes out in different directions. If you have a balloon that has all these little holes and punctures in it, even if it is a helium balloon, it will slowly fall to earth. It is the same with sexuality. If we keep depleting our resources we will have nothing left.

Second, sex is a need. It is like needing food – we need to be connected to another human being, we need to touch, you need to feel their heartbeat and the warmth of their skin. Masturbation weans us off that need, and it subverts the life instinct to actually want another person.

The biggest mistake that men and women make when entering into a new relationship is not to be completely romantic and look forward to a joyous life together. They minimise their expectations, and the result is that they rarely maximise the potential of their relationships. All of them enter into a new relationship expecting to maximise maybe 10 per cent of it, because they listen to the 'sexual experts' who say, 'You have to expect to argue, you should expect that there will be periods when you don't want to talk to each other…' So people enter into a relationship thinking that 10 per cent of what a relationship should be is the best they can get.

I think that the reason people are happy to settle for this 10 per cent is that they are too afraid to practise radical honesty. They fear exposure, and without this emotional nakedness, their relationship is going to suffer, and it will never reach the potential it innately has.

TIPS

1. READ MY BOOKS
2. Practise having sex with eyes open
3. Institute a period of sexual separation in your marriage
4. Never walk around the bedroom naked
5. Express all your sexual fantasies to your partner, especially well into marriage
6. Play erotic games during the relationship.

Winton Higgins

Winton Higgins was born in Sydney to a goldmining and grazing family in 1941. He grew up on a remote sheep station in central Australia. He has studied at the Universities of Sydney, Stockholm and London. His first career was law, his second was politics. He has lived in Sweden for extended periods, first as a graduate student, then as an academic researcher in politics.

He has been with his Swedish wife Lena for 21 years and they have two bilingual daughters.

Winton has been a practising Buddhist since 1987, and now teaches Buddhism and meditation at Wat Buddha Dhamma, a wilderness retreat centre north of Sydney, and at the Buddhist Library and Meditation Centre in Sydney.

He has researched and written about Buddhist sexual ethics and tolerance to help the community understand Buddhism.

As a Buddhist, I make no special effort to isolate sexuality as a privileged or problem area. On a wider view, what goes right and wrong in our sex lives follows the same pattern of satisfaction and dissatisfaction as our lives in general. Buddhist teaching and practice aims to understand and overcome suffering, and to pursue happiness, understood as freedom, as spiritual enlargement.

Taking up Buddhist practice has inordinately improved the quality of my life. It has given me a sense of personal authenticity and spaciousness, of knowing what I'm about. It gives full vent to my curiosity and love of investigation, while setting up clear priorities for me to live by. Clarity without closure! Naturally, when a gift like this falls into your lap, you want to share it, which is why I am now a Buddhist teacher.

One of the uses of Buddhism in the West is to subvert the messages we constantly get from our consumerist culture, what I call the Advertising Agency's View of the World. Just watch television ads – they tell us the more we consume, especially things we never thought of consuming before, the happier we'll be. Buddhism teaches the exact opposite – the more contentment we cultivate, the happier we'll be. In our culture sex itself has been turned into a sort of consumer item, like a car.

In the Advertiser's View of the World, if we aren't getting lots of varied sexual experience then we're missing out, we're losers, we're failures. This view distorts the fact that sex is a form of communication and a natural, and naturally limited, drive that needs to find its proper proportion in our complex and multifaceted lives.

When people on courses ask me questions about sex, I sense the sheer anxiety that the Advertiser's View of the World creates in them. Glossy mags are full of articles that ask 'Are You Getting Enough Sex?' and then tell you about some sex therapist's fantasy figures, which say you must ensure you get so many orgasms a week. This is the model, folks; conform or be a loser! Few things give me more satisfaction as a Buddhist teacher than showing students why this sort of obsessive-compulsive stuff is really, truly insane. It leads to the opposite of happiness, the opposite of freedom. Like all forms of insanity, it is excruciating and confining.

The actual mechanism of spiritual growth in Buddhism is learning to experience absolutely everything freshly, with 'a beginner's mind', as the Zen tradition puts it so well. Like so many others, I suppose, I have at various times found myself in sexual situations acting habitually, without the necessary freshness of attention, and above all insensitively to my partner.

To practise Buddhism is to have a message constantly flashing in front of your eyes: Lift Your Game! Not, of course, in a performance sense, but in the sense that we can always notice more, enter into our partner's experience more, be more aware of the consequences of what we're doing. Above all, this practice has made it painfully clear to me when my 'game' has been heading in the wrong direction, towards heedlessness.

Buddhism neither suppresses sexuality nor 'approves' of certain sexual practices and 'disapproves' of others. You can certainly find puritanical and prejudicial attitudes in some Buddhist countries and circles, but these attitudes arise from specific ethnic cultures, not from Buddhist doctrine. As I've already indicated, Buddhism seems to be unique among religions in denying that sex is a special problem that needs special rules. Rather, sex is an area in which we may have to redouble our efforts to apply general moral principles – love, non-harming, generosity, honesty and awareness.

The power of sexual desire calls forth a special precept – the third of five basic Buddhist precepts, whereby we undertake to avoid 'sexual misconduct'. But sexual misconduct doesn't refer to any particular sexual practice. Rather, it refers to sexual conduct based on greed, manipulation, dishonesty and violence.

In Western Buddhist centres you'll often find quite a few gays and lesbians. This is because Buddhism offers them a spiritual path that doesn't in any way make their sexual preference problematic. The line between sexual misconduct and being sexually responsible has nothing whatever to do with sexual preferences and technicalities.

I'm not sure there is such a thing as 'Buddhist philosophy' to help balance sexual and spiritual energy, as Buddhism is above all a practice. And as a practice, it would never bracket sexual and spiritual energy off from one another, and attempt to 'balance' them. As practitioners we're ideally on the job every second of the day.

Cultivating awareness of our sexual impulses, feelings, intentions, actions and experiences is a challenging aspect of spiritual practice. Making love doesn't constitute time out from spiritual practice; it may in fact be spiritually intense time in. All sorts of unforeseen personal challenges arise in bed!

But this practice would also challenge us to deal with any over-emphasis on sex in our lives. The Advertising Agency's view of sex as a consumer item, 'the more the better', is misleading, and so stupefying. Obsession is imprisonment for our intimates and us. The Buddhist practitioner has to continually ask her- or himself: am I giving enough priority to my daily meditation practice? Do I make time for intensive retreats? Am I honouring my non-sexual relationships and friendships (especially spiritual friendships)? Am I contributing to the personal development of my sexual partner(s), or am I being self-seeking, acquisitive and possessive?

EXERCISE: LEARNING TO APPRECIATE BEAUTY AND THEN LETTING IT GO

Many, perhaps most, people on intensive silent meditation retreats find themselves projecting intense longings and fantasies onto others. If I'm leading the retreat and sense that this may be arising for some participants, I suggest they try to refine their attention to see what is actually going on in separate stages. Buddhist practice is very investigative! At retreats, as in everyday life, we often catch sight of people with an arresting physical grace or beauty – commonly young, slim and with classical features.

Our first split-second response to this sight may be simply aesthetic appreciation, the same as when we see a beautiful butterfly suddenly cross our line of sight, or come over a rise and see an exquisite sunset. Have we developed our powers of inner observation sufficiently to see what comes in the next moment, when we lay a lot of knee-jerk stuff on top of that aesthetic appreciation – when we eroticise it, when the little acculturated voice inside screams: 'I've got to have it!'

We don't have to acquire, possess, conquer, consume or go to bed with the butterfly or the sunset to receive the blessing of its beauty. Why must we do it with people? Let's probe a bit instead. Just whose voice is that one of desperate longing? Who is thinking these thoughts?

I especially recommend this practice to men. Our sexuality is so visual, and we've often been brainwashed from birth to conquer and acquire everything that initially attracts us. Much of the time we'd enrich our own lives, and those of the women around us, by learning to cherish that first fleeting joy, and then skipping the rest of the drama. I never did understand the attraction of collecting a lot of dead butterflies pinned to a display board.

10

The Rhythm of Life Has A Powerful Beat

All the men in this book were asked their ideas and feelings on having a good relationship, monogamy and celibacy. Their life experiences have taken them on unique sexual journeys and I wanted to know what they had learnt about love, lust and living with and without sex. Their answers form a fascinating montage of opinions on these hot topics.

Having a good relationship

Many couples who come to me for counselling cannot express their love for each other. When I ask them what positive relationship role models they have had in their life they look at me blankly. Many of them say 'none'. They tell me that their parents did not have a good relationship, or that their mother always felt a certain amount of resentment towards their father.

I have often heard my clients say that they did not ever see their parents touch, or spend any time together. In short, they had no experience of seeing a good relationship and therefore found it difficult to create a healthy, loving connection of their own.

So the outcome of this sad reality is that most people don't know how to have a good relationship. Women's relationship books and magazines often blame men for this problem, portraying them as commitment-phobic, uncaring or just after as much easy sex as possible. Is this true? I don't think so. But what do men want in a relationship? Read on and the answers may surprise you.

Monogamy

The hottest topic I asked about was monogamy, and it was here that the differences between men and women became most starkly apparent.

For most women monogamy is, if not a non-issue, an issue

of little importance, in that they take it for granted that relationships should be monogamous. This was true whether they were monogamous or not. For the men I interviewed monogamy was a big issue, a fundamental issue within a relationship and one that was most often described as 'unnatural'.

Many of the men here believe that men are just not hardwired for monogamy, that it goes against the natural Darwinian idea that men need to spread their 'seed' far and wide in order to ensure that they have (plenty of) offspring.

Many men refused to countenance the idea of monogamy at all, believing it to be a societal construct that is anti-sexual freedom of choice. Even the men who had an emotional and intellectual commitment to monogamy in their relationships found it difficult, describing it as a struggle. To almost all of the men in this book it felt unnatural, even when it was a decision they had made freely.

This did not mean that the alternative was any easier and many spoke of the 'natural' male responses of jealousy and possessiveness towards their mate. Many men felt that the male ideal probably was a non-monogamous relationship free from jealousy. However, the difficulty in translating this to real life remained significant.

Celibacy

In a society that is sex obsessed, particularly for men, to abstain from sex is seen as a deeply radical, if sometimes abnormal, act. Celibacy still remains a touchy topic in the arena of sexuality.

Many men see celibacy as enforced by an anti-sexual pleasure culture, which says that if you are not married you should be celibate. The Church's dictate that those in religious orders should be celibate was criticised, even by those who see themselves as part of a traditional Church.

The men divided into those who claimed they would never voluntarily choose celibacy, and who saw it as a form of denial of the body, and those who saw 'time out' from sex as potentially sexually healing. This 'time out' allowed them to channel their powerful sexual energy into specific creative pursuits.

Men spoke of their sexual desire as being such a strong force in their life that to voluntarily abstain from sex allowed them to stop being controlled by it. Many men nominated focusing on their own spirituality as a time when they would voluntarily choose celibacy, as their sexual desire would be distracting.

Joseph Kramer

Having a good relationship

Men need to know that women go through times when they don't want to be penetrated. This doesn't mean that women don't want to be touched or don't want to be intimate; it just means they don't want to be penetrated.

Men and women need to know how to arouse themselves. A good relationship involves sharing your arousal with your partner. This knowledge of erotic arousal ideally should be learned at puberty. Our whole society would be transformed if only parents took time to prepare their children for that hormonal transformation called puberty. I suggest that boys and girls be encouraged and educated in the art of self-massage, including self-genital massage, for two years before puberty. Children need to be encouraged to honour and celebrate their bodies. Parents are responsible for giving their children a context for the radical changes that take place during puberty. This context often will involve the parents' religious beliefs. For example, 'Your body is created by God. Your sexuality is a gift from God. It is important to use this gift well and to be thankful for it.' Or perhaps, 'Pay attention to your capacity of pleasure and notice how your sexuality affects all of your relationships.' Certainly, the most appropriate sexual relationship for a pre-teen and teenager is with him- or herself. Most adults today are sexually wounded and incapable of authentic self-love because of the psychic, sexual abuse they experienced during puberty. Unfortunately, most pass this abusive, shameful experience on to their children.

Monogamy

I think of monogamy as one of the options for two folks to choose as the container for their relationship. It is a very special and powerful container. Some religions elevated this container to an exclusive status blessed by God. Thus monogamy was proclaimed the only moral option. I put being monogamous in the same category as living in a monastery or convent. It is difficult, glorious and not for most folks.

Celibacy

I am an expert on celibacy. When I was 17 years old I used to masturbate every day, but when I decided to enter the Jesuit novitiate, the rules were no sex, including masturbation. For three years I adhered to those rules. The celibacy seemed to activate other potentials within my personality. I was still very erotic, but my relationships were amazing for an 18 year old who lived as a sexual celibate.

Now, at 53, I am consciously celibate for weeks at a time. During these periods of no explicit sex, I pay attention to the many different expressions of sexuality in my being. The vibration is always there, so specific acts don't hold as much importance.

There are also times when I feel sexually content and satisfied. Excitement is an important element of my sexuality but contentment and bliss and satisfaction are equally important. I have taught 30–40 men and women a week how to touch and raise erotic energy, as well as having my own private massage practice, so for years I have been dancing in an erotic paradise. I have found that it is good for me to take a break and become a monk for a time, not out of desperation or fear, but to interrupt my patterns. This celibacy is not a negative reaction to explicit sex. It is just exploring another way of being.

Mantak Chia

Having a good relationship

It is important for people to love themselves and through this to be able to extend this love to their partner.

Central to my teaching is for couples to meditate together using the healing energy of compassion, combined with techniques of multi-orgasmic energy. This is a combination of breath and visualisation. The focus is for men to increase their yang or fire energy and women their yin or water energy. This leads to an energy exchange, as a woman's cooler water energy and a man's hot energy balance one another. I find that practising the Healing Love technique, which does not purely focus on the genitals but on redirecting orgasmic energy up the centre of the body to the top of the head and down again, can expand a couple's lovemaking and make a happier relationship.

In a same-sex relationship you need to create a yin–yang balance because one of the elements will be missing. This can be done because everyone is a combination of both yin and yang, it requires awareness.

Monogamy

Due to the intimate exchange of increased amounts of intense arousal energy during sex, partners have a strong effect on each other. Sexual energy has the property that it interacts with, and multiplies energy that it encounters within the body. It affects one's vital organs, emotions, mental state and spiritual condition. This can be good or bad. Multiplying negative energies will yield unpleasant after-effects. Both partners should learn to transform their negative energies on a daily basis, and especially before engaging in sex. By developing a mutually respectful, loving and trusting relationship, a deep bonding will result in the pleasureful ambience shared during and after sexual communion. This is best cultivated in a committed one-to-one relationship, monogamy.

Celibacy

Celibacy is the same as Tao practice: no ejaculation. In celibacy, you can massage the sexual organ, activating the sexual energy and drawing the energy up to the crown, so there is no need for sex itself, or for a partner. Sexual hormones need to reach the brain each day to maintain good health and good spiritual practice, but you can do this while celibate using Taoist techniques.

Stan Dale

Having a good relationship

The main ingredient is to love and accept yourself before you can do that with another human being. Relationships are not a 50–50 proposition; it is actually 200 per cent, 100 per cent being made up from each person. You need to be honest in your communication about how you feel about yourself. When you claim that another person has caused you to feel a certain way, maybe you just want to shift the blame. You need to do a lot of work on yourself before you can have a healthy relationship with another.

Monogamy

The way we are programmed by society leads to a lot of

misunderstandings. A man is a stud if he goes out and sleeps around, but this is not the way a woman is programmed, so when a man and woman become involved, often the man still wants to sleep around. This is not going to work for the couple unless they agree, and our entire society conspires against this.

Monogamy is a choice; the couple should carve this out together, without judgement. When the Human Awareness Institute took a survey, as many women as men were into non-monogamous relationships.

Celibacy

Most people have been programmed that sex is intercourse, but if you accept sex as a sacred energy exchange, then why would I want celibacy?

Celibacy is a choice. I might not choose to be sexual with myself or another for a short or long period of time, but it's always personal and nothing to do with anyone else's vision of you. I was in the desert for three months and I decided to play with my sexuality. Sometimes the decision was to be sexual with myself and other times I was celibate for a few weeks at a time. When you choose, do something that is positive for yourself, instead of destructive. There can be a lot of growth.

Willem de Ridder

Having a good relationship

Science has known already for quite some time that there is only energy in the universe. You and I are pure energy. In fact we're ONE. There is nothing wrong with being alone, but 'the lonely crowd' is the highest cause of death in big cities, because if you drop anybody, you are dropping yourself. We are raised in the West with the opposite idea, that we're all separated. We have learned that others can think about us. So we're terrified of what others think about us. We behave, act normal, make good impressions, dress up, be interesting, beautiful, intelligent, etc, etc. We get very angry when somebody else fails to do so.

So if we don't like that somebody, we have a terrible feeling. We blame her for that horrible feeling we have, but don't want. We can't help it. We're powerless. We have given her all the power. She can give us a terrible feeling... That's what we've learned. But we're far from powerless. We can in fact think what we want. The moment I see others as perfect human beings my whole world opens up. Sexuality is stopped through you being demanding in relationships (you have to be nice, otherwise I can't love you).

Our thoughts are very powerful. They create our (so-called) reality. If I think you're terrible, I see a terrible person. I create you. It's that simple. If I am convinced that the city is dangerous, there is a good chance that something horrible will happen there. We have great power. We can create what we want. Just try it. If you say you are alone, then the entire universe will support you in that. If you treat your enemy as a friend he will soon become one. To have a good relationship, I have to realise that I have no power over others – the only thing I can do is to make it great for myself.

If you see in your partner things you don't like, you have to realise that there is no way you can change things there. Somebody else might see different qualities in your partner, so who is right? All you see is yourself! You are the one who's seeing, feeling, experiencing and reacting. It's all happening in your own body. You can take your power back very easily. If you are sure that your partner makes you feel horrible, try to feel that feeling and for a moment don't call it 'horrible' or give it any other name. Don't even connect your partner with that feeling. Just the feeling itself. Disconnected from any thoughts.

Feelings don't think. You're the one that will glue a label on it. The moment you give a name to a feeling, they're both stuck together for the rest of your life. It stagnates everything. Since your body wants to stream with sexual energy, it warns you with an uncomfortable feeling. We project that feeling on our partner. We blame her or him. If you let all stories and labels go for a moment and accept that feeling wholeheartedly, embrace it and love yourself doing it, you liberate the feeling from the label you connected to it. They both start streaming again and gone is that horrible feeling and memory. You start seeing a totally different partner. It's like a miracle... You have to get used to it. That's why I wanted to start that Sex School many years ago [see Chapter 2].

I wrote a book about it called *Handbook of Mirrorology*. It tells you all about your great power that you can only grab back if you start practising with some other people. You cannot do this on your own. The book is already in its third printing and about one thousand little 'fanclubs' are joining weekly to practise with each other. Incredible miracles are happening instantly. Your body wants this desperately. If you give it one finger it immediately takes the whole hand. Sexual and emotional tenderness leads to great pleasure. Then you become aware that it all starts with you.

The only way that sex and life start to move is for you to start giving freely. By opening up to the others and giving them trust, you actually are giving it to yourself. Only by giving, you get things back; if you wait until somebody will be nice to you, you can wait forever.

Monogamy

The Chinese marriage used to be quite different to the Western one. In China a marriage was a kettle with cold water, which was then put on the fire. In the West the marriage was a kettle with boiling water, taken off the fire. Most Western relationships seem to cool off after a hot start. Women are told that men are always horny when they see a beauty. But the truth is different. As I told before, it is the woman who radiates sexual energy that triggers men. A woman just has to look a certain way, and soon a man will be begging for her favours. Most women don't know this and blame men for their effects or their negation of female power. The longer you are together, the more energy will grow and bloom if you let it, which can lead to incredible experiences. To walk out, you lose everything and have to start all over again. From scratch. The question is if you will ever reach that high level again. To be monogamous can be more difficult for a man if he is unaware that another femme fatale has focused her power on him and he becomes wax in her hands. Most men are afraid of women. That's why they suppressed them for so long.

Celibacy

Sexuality is not just the act of penetration and spilling the beans. It is the pure energy that supports us completely, if we dare to open our heart to it. Even if you don't have any physical sex, it is still very important to be totally open to everybody, or at least to someone. If you are celibate, because you have no real energy contact with anybody, your body suffers. Since the entire universe is pure energy, we are energy too. So in fact there is no difference between you and me. [If you are celibate,] not only does your body suffer, its life force deteriorates.

If your heart is open to everybody, your body feels very satisfied and functions perfectly, even if you are alone. If you are with a partner, the contact can be so intense that even without physical sex life can be heaven. It is important to touch and be touched. That's why many lonely people have pets. In orphanages they discovered that babies who weren't touched at all simply died.

Keith Hennessy

Having a good relationship

We all want love. We all want to be with someone or someones. I consider this to be one of life's great struggles. There is no answer, only practice. It is an honour to practise loving and to practise opening yourself to loving. Marco Vassi writes of three complementary sexual expressions: monogamy, promiscuity and celibacy. Each of us will braid these three paths differently at various times in our lives.

Monogamy

When describing a relationship of sexual exclusiveness I tend not to use the term 'monogamy' because it seems too full of projections, assumptions and judgements. Likewise I don't use the words 'non-monogamy' or 'promiscuity' because they tend to be inarticulate labels applied by an external perspective, rather than a self-definition by experimental sex radicals.

My home base is a sex-positive, queerlicious culture, which honours honesty more than monogamy, and ecstasy more than control. Held in the loving arms of this intentionally perverse embrace I have often chosen to be sexually exclusive with one man. I have done this to fulfil two complementary goals.

First, to create a container of intimate trust in the early phase of a relationship. Letting my boyfriend know that I intend to focus only on him provides all kinds of indescribable freedoms, especially if either partner has a tendency towards jealousy, or has been sexually betrayed.

Second, to create closed circuits of fluid exchange, a relatively safe practice of conscious, non-condomed sex. During these periods of exclusivity I have continued to facilitate rituals of ecstasy and intimacy with groups of naked men, and sometimes women; I have continued to fantasise while jerking off; and I have continued a creative practice of physical performance, exploration and intense human contact. These practices provide some outlet for the parts of me that want to make love with the whole world whenever I feel like it.

Celibacy

Celibacy, both in despair and by intention, has been very important to my sexual healing and creative emergence. There is so much to explore and unlearn. It takes time to study our sexual impulses, fantasies, ideas and potential. How do we know what we really want? In my experience it's emotionally, physically and psychically rewarding to take time not pursuing sex and love with others. I have relied on lengthy periods of celibacy – one or two years – to recover from intense relationships and prepare for the next.

I've also experimented with shorter periods of what I might call classical celibacy, no sex including with myself, sometimes to build energy for a lover, other times just to clear myself from an obsessive phase of fantasising. From the ages of 25 to 28 I was relationship-celibate: that is how I refer to a period of self-discovery in which I didn't have sex with anyone. I did however learn to truly enjoy having sex with the world and myself.

I became a sexual pagan, in love with the earth, enamoured by trees, lustful of the sun and seduced by the ocean. My animal and spiritual natures were revealed in lengthy solosex rituals. I discovered the intense pleasure hiding at the root of my dick, buried a few inches up my bum. I read copiously, something I never have time to do when I'm with a lover. I studied sexual liberation, queer histories, feminist spirituality, the anatomy of pleasure (a Carol Queen term) and the relationship between sexual fantasy, archetypal psychology and myth.

I read lots of porn, noticing patterns of what turned me on, what scared me and what made me upset. I came to my own conclusions about sexist, racist, ageist and other forms of hurtful images. I read some Taoist guides and I practised not-cumming. I experimented with the alchemy of sexual energy, the power of a yin or non-ejaculation orgasm and I learnt that sex could be a prayer. In the alleged prime of youth I lived as a private celibate in one of the world's most erotic cities and there I discovered myself as a polysexual animal in love with the world.

As for the culture in relation to celibacy, the culture is mean. We are shamed for being alone and teased by all kinds of bullies, including advertising and Hollywood, if we don't have that special someone. But these industries profit greatly from making us feel ugly, stinky and generally not sexy. Not to mention that most Euro- and American-based cultures are addicted to speed and productivity, which is the worst environment for contemplation, revelation and intimacy. So let's not worry too much that there's no respect from mainstream cultures for a diversity of sexual expression, which includes celibacy.

Panos Couros

Having a good relationship
I believe in Kahlil Gibran's words about marriage:

> Love one another, but make not a bond of love: Let it rather be a moving sea between the shores of your souls. Fill each other's cup but drink not from one cup. Give one another of your bread but eat not from the same loaf. Sing and dance together and be joyous, but let each one of you be alone. Even as the strings of a lute are alone though they quiver with the same music. Give your hearts, but not into each other's keeping. For only the hand of Life can contain your hearts. And stand together yet not too near together: For the pillars of the temple stand apart, and the oak tree and the cypress grow not in each other's shadow.

What I have learnt is this: be tactful, be honest, don't wear the other person's shit, don't buy into issues that are theirs, not yours and learn that being 'in love' is often being 'in need'. In a relationship always question the nature of your actions and your motivations – are you acting out of love, or because you want a certain response from your partner?

Never give up your personal space and always have your own refuge, which is yours alone, and always love yourself more than your partner. Ultimately we are all alone, and if you are not at peace with that you can't come together and make a life together with anyone.

Monogamy

The only way I can be monogamous is my way. When I am committed to someone I am monogamous with my heart and with my expression of intimacy, but not with my body. My body I share! When I am in a loving relationship I hold a part of my heart and spirit exclusively for my lover, no one can go there but them, but that doesn't mean that I can't be sexual with another person.

Emotional commitment does not equal sexual monogamy and my heart life is different to my sexual activities. Basically men are designed to spawn, so spawn I must and spawn I do.

Celibacy

Celibacy is hard in this society; you are damned if you choose it and damned if you don't. Sex isn't everything. Sometimes, in order to achieve a high level of spiritual awareness, the vibrational energy of sexuality is disruptive and irrelevant. When you are in a deep meditative state, not being actively sexual is of benefit. Celibacy is an option to choose. People shouldn't be sexually pressured because this just makes sex a big issue, which it shouldn't be.

Shai Shahar

Having a good relationship
You know, I read somewhere that any man who wouldn't lie to his woman had no regard for her feelings. It's an interesting idea. I guess women can understand certain lies men tell, but most would rather we conducted ourselves in ways such as we wouldn't have to lie. Therefore it is important to tell the truth, the whole truth and nothing but the truth on the very first day of the relationship. The truth about your sexual proclivities, attractions, habits, history, fantasy and desires in this brand new relationship. That way, when she catches you with the other woman she won't be able to say it's your fault.

No, really, you get very few chances to get it right in life, so if you want quality and bonding you better be honest with yourself and her. Learn to compromise and to sexually include her wishes within yours. When you communicate do your best to be positive – no sarcasm, no insults, EVER, but that doesn't mean you can't argue, or won't. Play games, go outdoors and explore a lot, seduce others as a couple once in a while. And remember, only the one who hurts you can make it better.

Monogamy
The closest I ever came to 'monogamous' was in a Scrabble game, and when I was married, but even then my wife and I explored ourselves sexually with a couple of couples, so I guess it's how you view things.

I am currently delightfully bonded to, and with, a wonderfully polyamorous, green-eyed vixen, sexual healer, adventurer and co-conspirator called Cora, who shares my view that bodies were meant to share. Having said that, it was wonderful to go back to having sex without a condom again.

Celibacy

I never judge any situation, even if I don't agree with it. As long as one's celibacy is voluntary and not mandatory or enforced I have no issue with it. And sure, I can understand a bit of abstinence making the heart grow fonder. The problem comes when celibacy is the result of a fanatically held notion that sex is dirty and that wanting to have sex, or someone wanting to have sex with you, makes you dirty.

Some have the idea that sex brings complications to an otherwise simple life, but to me that is like saying mayonnaise brings complications to an otherwise simple chicken sandwich. On the other hand, with AIDS and the strange behaviour of strangers once you've had sex with them, the thought had crossed my mind that maybe I'd wait for the 'right girl' to come along, but that's not celibacy, is it? Anyway, in the end there were too many of them.

Dan Savage

Having a good relationship

First decide whether you want to have a purely asexual relationship, or a long-term relationship. A long-term relationship, or marriage, can become something more than sex, and sex itself can fade in importance. That is OK.

A lot of perfectly good relationships are ended because they have become non-sexual and people feel it is not a real relationship any more, and that they need to find someone else. Maybe people should stay together and get those physical needs met outside the relationship, while having their primary intimate needs met inside the relationship, but this is not talked about in our culture because people don't feel comfortable with it.

Men tend to be kinkier than women and you can't just will their fetishisms away. This is something that you need to incorporate into your sex life, because if you can't give him permission to do it with you then he will do it behind your back.

Monogamy
Women should be realistic about men's sexual behaviour, as they have not been evolved for monogamous behaviour. Women's sexuality acts as a check on male heterosexual licence. It is much more difficult for men to get laid. In gay culture it is the opposite and it is too easy for gay men to get laid.

If you look at the behaviour of all the other male mammals on the planet, most of them are all aggressively seeking sex, while the female is not being so receptive to sex. There are also studies on female non-monogamy that show that human sperm competes with other sperm, the assumption being that a female will have more than one sexual partner.

Celibacy
Permissiveness is not only the permission to have sex, but the permission not to have sex. If you desire not to be sexually active then more power to you. I do think that there is too much pressure in our culture, which makes people feel like there is something wrong with them if they are not having sex, or taking a break from sex. This is not true. It should always be about what makes you happy and content. If sex makes you miserable don't have it, and if being alone gives you more energy, or you get more work done and are therefore more content, this works for you.

Everyone wants to take what works for them and project it onto everyone else. You then have people saying sex three times a week works for me, then it must be the same for everyone else. If everyone does what feels right for them, whether it is being sexually active or not, people would be so much happier.

Justin Case

Having a good relationship

I would have to say that having a gender transition in a relationship is not the ideal ingredient for making life easy. However, I think that the skills my partner and I had to use to survive my gender transition were good communication, honesty and the ability to focus on the big issues, not obsess on the details. This is what makes for a very successful relationship. The other thing I think it is important to remember when you are in a relationship is that you are IN a relationship, you are not the centre of the relationship.

Monogamy

I think that monogamy or non-monogamy is, like everything else, something to be discussed and negotiated for each relationship. It should not be some unspoken assumption. In my sexual relationship experience monogamy has been appropriate at times, while at other times non-monogamy was right. I have had relationships of each type and some where it has shifted in the relationship, by consent and after discussion. When I started taking testosterone my sex drive certainly increased, but my value system and belief in open communication did not change.

Celibacy

I think celibacy is as valid a sexual choice as any other form of consenting sexuality. In a relationship I think that, like any other type of sexuality, it is something that both parties would have to want. There is a lot of pressure on men to be sexual all the time and to be able to 'get it up' on cue. Sex is fun, but it is not all there is to a relationship. Having said that, I can't imagine a time when I would want to be celibate, but I suppose many people can't imagine wanting to try SM either.

Richard Pacheco

Having a good relationship

If you prize intimacy then you need to reveal the truth. When my wife and I met, it was the second time around for both of us. We had been in relationships that had failed because of jealousy and an inability to cope with multiple partners. When we met and fell in love we agreed that we would be engaged in the telling of the truth, because if we were going to lie to one another and feel betrayal that would only produce madness and chaos. There were plenty of painful times, but our relationship has endured because of our willingness to keep trying and keep connecting. We have been together since 1971.

Monogamy

Marlon Brando once said, 'I don't think it's the nature of any man to be monogamous. Men are propelled by genetically ordained impulses over which they have no control to distribute their seed.'

And while one could easily argue the point about a man's actual ability to control the urge to distribute his seed, I, like many another married man, have certainly had the occasion to resent the need for such an exercise.

Celibacy

In my world, celibacy is something I just don't get. Our bodies offer us an incredible gift of pleasure, and after breathing and eating, sex provides my idea of a good day. I feel like a lot of people, when they have sexual problems and trauma, rather than face them and work their way through them, just turn themselves off. Often there is a lot of redirected sexual energy, leading to all sorts of convoluted mischief. I think that sexually active and healthy people make the world a much more fun place to call home.

Jack Heidenry

Having a good relationship and monogamy

A good sexual relationship, especially a monogamous one, is also a sexual ideal, and probably the percentage of people who fall short of it is about the same as celibates who fail; but at least it is a worthy ideal, and not an anti-sexual one. I personally think that all sexual relationships should be monogamous, which may not be perfect, but it's better than anything else around. Swinging may be OK for a few, probably the same as for an open marriage, and various other non-monogamous sexual lifestyles, but in my opinion they never work in the long run, and it's usually the woman who gets the short end of the sexual stick.

Men will go along with any sexual opportunity that gives them access to more rather than only one woman, and if the woman goes along with that she's being a sap. If a woman gives her body to a man, she has a right to demand that their relationship be exclusive. Monogamy is difficult for men – their genetic instinct is to lay as many women as possible – but the survival of the family, which is what the human race is based on, is ultimately dependent on a core unit of a woman, a man and offspring.

Men, and now women, are also responsible for raising children, and the main cause of a broken home and unhappy children just happens to be that either the man or woman decided not to be monogamous. Not that I'm against divorce, by the way. Divorce can be good, healthy, even necessary at times; but I think cheating on your partner is plain wrong. No amount of sexual sophistication can ever replace common sense.

Celibacy

I have taken numerous potshots at so-called sex advice people. The only thing I will say is that the sex advice industry is not only run by mediocrities, but its main goal is to get people to overachieve sexually. Couples (or individuals) should feel free and under no pressure to do or be anything other than what they want to be sexually, whether that means celibacy, fetishism, monogamy or whatever, and at whatever level that suits them.

A lot of people go through periods of celibacy, or more specifically, abstinence. Celibacy implies a lifestyle, whereas abstinence implies a sexual relationship from which somebody is taking either a voluntary or enforced vacation. Celibacy as a vocation is perfectly valid, so long as it is not held up, as it has been in the Christian Church for millennia, as a higher and more perfect state than marriage. The anti-sexual overtones that derive from the superiority complex of celibates have resulted in much of Christianity's heritage as an anti-sex religion. (Of course, the Church does affirm sexuality as a sacrament in the context of marriage, so it is not entirely anti-sexual.)

A friend of mine, Bob Francoeur, who is the author of about 22 books on sex, has spent a lot of time studying various new sexual lifestyles that are emerging as people adapt to their life situations. He is also a former priest. Anyway, he knows many priests and nuns who are unwilling to give up their religious vocations because they enjoy the spiritual life and a life of service to others. However, they hate the celibacy, so they have sexual relationships with women or men, as the case may be, of like mind. This isn't hypocrisy, it's a Darwinian adaptation. Celibacy is falling apart at the seams – nobody practises pure and perfect celibacy and probably nobody ever has.

Homosexuality is rampant in so-called 'celibate' priesthoods, with some estimates at up to 75 per cent. I edited a book not long ago (see theposition.com for an excerpt) on the sex life of nuns, and the amazing thing is that so many nuns masturbated (the book was written by an ex-nun as her doctoral thesis). In short, celibacy is imperfect both as an ideal and as practice – it's anti-sexual and unworkable.

Robbie Swan

Having a good relationship
I don't know that I am qualified to speak on this really. My relationship with Fiona has been the best one of my life and the real difference in it from the others has been the openness about sex and about one's feelings for having sex.

Monogamy
Once you admit to each other that monogamy is not the important thing in the relationship but love and honesty are... something happens. I think it's got to do with the fact that very few of us are monogamous beings and that almost everyone fantasises or lusts after another person at some time. My experience is that as soon as you can be totally honest about this, and prepared to discuss it at a level and frequency commensurate with the importance that sex holds in your relationship, you become liberated from all the usual suspects that assist relationship breakdown – jealousy, envy, lust, etc.

Celibacy
To be a natural celibate is not to lose sight of your sexuality, but is fused with your awareness. Sex is not there for pleasure, but procreation, but for most people sex brings enormous amounts of pleasure, be it physical or emotional. And most people need it. I think if celibacy is forced on you by someone else it does the most incredible psychological and spiritual damage.

Layne Winklebleck

Having a good relationship
The key element in a relationship, which maximises the ability of the partners to achieve their highest vision of themselves, is spontaneity. Sometimes partners in a relationship instinctively

struggle to move the relationship in the opposite direction, towards predictability. Partners try to teach the other how to behave in order to meet expectations.

Counsellors and therapists sometimes teach negotiation as a means for smoothing things out, but sometimes the smoother things get the more stagnant and boring they get. In no area is this truer than in sex. Sexual desires are a moving target. We get bored with doing the same old thing over time and need to feel free to experiment. We need to be able to be whimsical and playful.

Monogamy

Kat, my wife, and I are not monogamous, or possessive, or jealous and have never been during our 20 (God what is it now) 2 [year] or so relationship. We have both had many lovers and play partners and playthings. I don't really understand monogamy. Would it be difficult? Sure seems like it would. Yup. Sure does.

Celibacy

I never really asked for my sexuality, actually. I certainly did not become a sexual slut because it was a role expectation of my cultural group. Testosterone-driven demons grabbed me by the dick during adolescence and shook me every which way but loose. No complaints. Loved every minute of it.

But now that I'm 62, golf is starting a serious competition for my daydreams and I've got no complaints about that either. I followed my bliss sexually when it was big for me and I'm still generally following my bliss, except now tomato plants are big. Same way with couples, is the way I look at it. If we think we have a problem because we are supposed to be sexual, but we don't much feel like it, that really misses the point.

Robert McGinley

Having a good relationship

Respect is essential, not only for the other but for oneself. One cannot be a dependent person and have a good relationship. Your happiness cannot come from someone else making you happy; it has to come from you.

Monogamy

Swinging is monogamous because you are married to one person. It's about being open and honest and being in agreement with one's partner. I disagree with sexual cheating, which is dishonestly going behind your partner's back for sex with someone else.

Celibacy

There are phases of our lives and changes. It could be that we need to heal a break-up of a relationship through not having sex, or we use this time to sexually experiment.

David Steinberg

Having a good relationship

This is one of the great philosophical issues of all time.

Monogamy

As for monogamy, I think it's essentially problematic and unnatural, which is why so few people practise it in fact, although a lot of people give lip service to it in theory. The dominant paradigm for sex in couples today is not monogamy, it's multiple sexual relationships in the form of secret, guilt-ridden affairs.

On the other hand, open, honest non-monogamy is tremendously demanding of people in terms of trust, ego issues and complex understanding of how sexual energy really works and what that does and does not mean. I don't think many couples are equipped to handle the real stresses of honest non-monogamy, and maybe secret affairs are as good as it gets for those people. Issues of jealousy, sexual insecurity, sexual incompatibility and so on don't go away when people declare themselves to be monogamous – they just go underground.

Celibacy

I can't say I've felt this very much myself, but I think it's as important to respect the desire not to be sexual as it is to respect the desire to be sexual. Men in particular are taught that they should want sex all the time, the more the better, but it's not really the way it works for any of the hundreds of men I've spoken with and counselled over the years.

Although we try to deny it, sex is vulnerable for everyone, and only a fool would want to be vulnerable all the time, with people they don't know or people they don't have any reason to trust. The body knows this even when the mind wants to deny it, which is why a lot of men's bodies run the other way in certain sexual situations.

Kenneth Ray Stubbs

Having a good relationship

I do not understand relationships, and I don't think anyone does. I have never wanted to be married, but I have been in relationships. What I know about sexuality and sensuality is: don't play any games and don't behave like a robot. Forget the theory that men are from Mars and women are from Venus, it is perhaps the biggest pile of bullshit in our human belief drama.

Monogamy

I suspect that many men and many women have natural proclivities towards both monogamy and multiple-partner behaviour and emotions. I would hold these proclivities to be genetically based, with various cultural influences functioning as powerful parameters.

Again, my main point is the fallacy in the male–female dichotomy. Fortunately, the concept of 'intersex' is starting to be embraced in Western sexology. Do you know for sure that your sex chromosomes are XX? Or XY? And even if they are, there are many, many variations in anatomy and temperament from individual to individual.

Celibacy

Wherever we are sexually I think it is very important to give ourselves permission to explore all the possibilities. There are shifts and changes that go on in our lives. The problem is often in long-term sexual relationships when one person does not feel like being sexual. It's important to be open and honest with how we feel about that relationship. I think that we need to trust our inner voice, just to observe and trust the process and give ourselves space. That can be very hard on our partner but if you do something against yourself it just robs you of your energy.

If we go through big life changes, such as a change in sexual orientation, or simply not feeling sexual, celibacy is an absolutely valid response to this. Celibacy is also about personal freedom, which needs to be honoured.

Kerry Riley

Having a good relationship

Some of the ingredients that have helped us are: Diane and I give our relationship high priority. We have decided to maintain sexual passion and a loving bond throughout our lives together, so we put a lot of time and energy into our relationship. We treat it as a very special entity. It is more important than each of our individual egos. It's something we work on as teammates, continually creating more and more love in our lives. It takes something more powerful than hoping, wishing or desiring. It takes a lifetime commitment.

We see the path of our relationship as one of the biggest paths to our own growth, and our fulfilment physically, spiritually, sexually. We see our relationship as a vehicle through which we get a tangible experience of love. For this reason she and I have decided to put a lot of energy, care and attention into it so we experience more love in this lifetime. We know at the end of our lives what will count more than everything else will be how much we loved.

The first thing to having a good relationship is the understanding that disharmony is part of a healthy relationship. Many people have the attitude that a good relationship must always be smooth and in control, so they aren't happy if that marriage doesn't happen like that. Knowing that joys and hurts are part and parcel of falling in love, the secret is to see them as a natural part of a healthy relationship. So understanding this we have practical ways we've developed for creating harmony again when we are out of sync. Instead of blaming each other or the relationship we use harmonising processes to get back on track with each other:

- *Communication.* Having ways of communicating what you like and what you don't like without making the other person feel that you are blaming them.
- *Keep your sex happening.* This is important; making a time, planning romantic holidays or nights away from home for making love, for telling your partner what touches your heart, for communicating what you love and appreciate about them and for having fabulous sex.

- *Explore the extraordinary in your lovemaking.* We see sex as the fuel of a passionate relationship. By studying the teaching of sacred sex you will discover [that] the ways you [can] make love are unlimited. Most couples never take time to explore any more than the patterns that work for them.

Monogamy

People need to work out between them agreements that work. If you have a deep, loving relationship you can communicate your desire to have interaction with others, but that doesn't necessarily mean intercourse. It can be a sexual connection dancing with another person and I am sure most couples would agree that it is OK for their partner to dance with someone else. Maybe it is OK to massage someone else, someone else's shoulders, but not OK to give them a whole body massage. But maybe it is OK if you both massage that person, having fun together giving that other person pleasure. Again, it doesn't need to involve intercourse.

If you want to explore the extraordinary together, you will need to be prepared to experiment. First I suggest you set boundaries, ground rules. What is OK, what is not OK, what you're prepared to experiment with before going into any sexual encounter. Always take the requests of the most conservative partner as the ground rules each time you experiment. After the encounter, allow time for the experience to settle, for the reactions to surface and subside before going further. If you love your partner, you have compassion and sensitivity for their needs as well as your own. Then as teammates on a journey into love together, you will work it out.

Celibacy

I chose a period of celibacy when I was in my late twenties. I was depleted from my trips to India and I was told by a healer that I could regenerate my vital energy through celibacy. I was so sick I didn't feel like sex much anyway, but it worried me because prior to my illness I wanted sex almost every day. Celibacy is something I tried as a last straw. However, the benefits surprised me. As a young person with high testosterone levels, whenever I met a woman I'd be thinking about sex. Now was an opportunity to meet women on all other levels. I discovered I really liked women, in fact I mostly mixed with women. I found their conversations far more encompassing and intimate than those of my mates. A whole new world opened for me; I discovered women for the first time. It was a time of inner growth, of discovery, of healing. What else was amazing was instead of always chasing women, something in my energy was now attracting women to me. Sex was available everywhere and ironically I was celibate.

Celibacy in a relationship is much more complicated, especially if one partner wants to try it but the other doesn't, there is a difference in desire or there is a physical problem like an erection dysfunction in a man or the woman feels little pleasure from intercourse. So one partner tells the other, 'I don't want sex' and this can destroy a relationship.

What is important is how you define sex. We need to expand our definition of sex. To many people sex equals intercourse, that's it. However, if we can see sex as a way of expressing love and sharing sexual energy, then that gives us a much wider choice than simply intercourse. There are lots of ways a couple can have sexual intimacy without intercourse. For many people, if they don't have intercourse, they don't have anything.

When a person doesn't want sex in a relationship it is important to take a deeper look and find out why. Is it physical, is it stress, is it health, is it that they are not feeling loved or appreciated, or not feeling emotionally nurtured? Whatever it is, you can learn ways to use your sexual love as healing, as energising, as a way of sharing love with your partner, other than just intercourse. Then there is a big chance that you will be able to work it out so that both partners' needs are met. Any man who has practised tantra knows that sexual loving can still happen in numerous ways, as it opens up trust.

Dr Jules Black

Having a good relationship

You have to think about marriage in this way: if we started a club, and one in two members were resigning, we would have to rethink the rules and objectives of our club. Well, the same thing is happening in marriage.

Monogamy

There is a joke about a husband and wife visiting the Royal Easter Show. They are going through the cattle pavilion and they see the various prize-winning bulls. Under the sign saying 'third prize', it says '100 services a year', and the wife says, 'Look at that'. They move on to the second prize winner, which says '150 services a year'. Then they come to the grand prize winner and it says '320 services a year', and the wife says, 'Wow, look at that!' and the husband says, 'But that bull gets a new cow every time'.

I believe it is difficult for men to be monogamous, as people are living so much longer. How can you maintain the same amount of enthusiasm and ardour and interest in the same partner? When I hear a man say, 'I am just as much in love with my wife as the day I married her 35 years ago', it sounds very nice, but I think he is stretching the truth.

Celibacy

It is becoming trendy to live in a sexually dysfunctional marriage, where the executive husband adorns his wife with clothes and jewels, and takes her to lovely places, but they never have sex because he is always too busy. It is all too common and the wives complain to me.

David Brown

Having a good relationship

There are three key facets to establishing a long-term relationship: understanding the true nature of love; discovering the power of agreement together; and developing the art of true communication.

When Jane and I first married, almost 30 years ago, I made a decision to agree to agree together. In other words my first act of agreement was to decide that issues within my relationship and my family would not become subject to my disagreements. This means that in the early years of my marriage we had to spend considerable periods of time discussing the different perspectives we had and because of our agreement to agree I would work at those issues until I reached an agreement together we could live with.

Agreeing to agree extends to agreeing with one another in the absence of the other as well as in the presence of your partner. This means that you can be certain that whether together or apart your partner is not speaking badly of you, or disagreeing with you behind your back. This builds an atmosphere of trust.

True communication means communicating your feelings to your partner and coming to understand their feelings so that you can endeavour to act in ways to help each other to move forward and not suffer needless hurt. This means the sharing of yourself and a willingness to be vulnerable with one another.

If you are in a current relationship that has 'run aground' or become 'dry' or within which you have begun experiencing sexual difficulties, then what you are learning about yourself and how to change is also going to require changes in your partner. You will need your partner to change her responses to you and to break some set patterns that you have found yourselves in. These changes cannot come about unless your partner is aware of the changes that are taking place in you and unless a change of heart is happening for both of you.

The responsibility for these inward changes to take place within your relationship rests with you. You have become aware of changes within yourself and to revert to old ways of thinking and acting within your relationship, especially within the intimate and sexual aspects, would be a betrayal of yourself and of your partner.

The big challenge now, however, is how do you communicate your current true feelings to your partner without evoking hostility and in a way that will effect a positive heart response from them?

Monogamy

My personal experience and viewpoint after 30 years of marriage is that:

- relationships are 'made in heaven';
- monogamous relationships are the ideal;
- a whole lifetime is insufficient time to fully perfect one heterosexual relationship;
- monogamous marriage is the most secure basis for children to be born into;
- monogamy is a matter of commitment and love rather than sexuality.

It is neither easier nor harder for men to be monogamous than women, but in general, men are not as good at maintaining sexual self-discipline as women.

Celibacy

In my opinion, celibacy would be a lifestyle adopted by an individual as a result of a vocation, eg a monk, a nun or someone in a similar religious order. I think in such circumstances the motivation and fulfilment that comes from a feeling of true self-worth within the structure of the vocation would mean that the individual is fulfilled enough without the necessity for sexual fulfilment. In such cases celibacy shouldn't be viewed as anything negative, or that the individual is deprived in any way, but on the contrary that he or she is privileged to be fully immersed and fulfilled in the context of their vocation.

I don't believe that a single person who is simply without relationships is in the same sense celibate. In such cases a single person may go for a long period of time, or possibly a whole lifetime, without fulfilling their sexuality with another, but this doesn't make them celibate. This could be the result of sexual repression, deprivation, isolation or a whole series of other such factors. In such circumstances an individual can learn to be in touch with his or her sexuality, and even be deeply fulfilled, in acts of self-loving and self-pleasuring. This may or may not be a perfect substitute for intimacy with another person, but is a more positive alternative than repression or deprivation.

There may be other career circumstances that would require someone to focus totally on the work that they do and as a result, and for the sake of that work, to leave aside issues that they regard as secondary, notably their sexuality.

A couple within a relationship who go through periods of non-sexual contact or feelings are not necessarily celibate. Non-sexual periods of time within a relationship may last from days to years and may be caused by a number of situations. For example, sickness and ill-health in one or both partners of the relationship, times of grief or spiritual contemplation can all cause sexuality to be temporarily inappropriate.

During such times it is imperative for the couple to maintain open and honest communication with each other. Relationships are ill-equipped to withstand periods of sexual abstinence, but not many relationships can endure emotional isolation for too long without suffering. Other couples run into a stage of their relationship where they may think that celibacy is their only option, for example when dealing with ageing. However, if the couple can understand that the foundation of all sexuality is intimacy, then they can continue to enjoy a sexual relationship throughout their lifetime.

Michael Castleman

Having a good relationship

What makes a great relationship? You have to like the person, love the person and be in love with the person. You need all three. If you only have two – and certainly if you only have one – things eventually don't work. You have to like the person as a friend, confidant, supporter, sounding board; a person who shares your values and a reasonable proportion of your interests.

You have to love the person, deeply care for their wellbeing and be willing to make sacrifices to maintain and nurture it. And you have to be in love with the person. There has to be sexual chemistry. Beyond that, I would say: two sinks in the bathroom. One separate vacation a year. Similar views about housekeeping. And cordial relations with the in-laws.

A good sexual relationship is a deep friendship between two people who are also lovers. But friendship – and beyond that, love – is ultimately more important than the sex. After all, even if you have sex daily (which very few long-term lovers do), that involves maybe an hour or two. But you spend much more time with the person out of bed. Generally, if time spent together out of bed isn't much fun, then the sex won't be much fun. So I'd say, look for a person you can be friends with.

Someone whose company you enjoy, who shares some of your interests, but also can introduce you to new ones, someone who has a good sense of humour, someone who can listen well, give you good feedback about issues you care about, someone who is kind, compassionate, appropriately flexible and appropriately assertive. And then someone who turns you on sexually.

Many men in long-term relationships get upset about the decline in sex after the first year or so, and envy single men or divorced men who, they imagine, get more sex. But all the surveys show that this is not the case. Single and divorced men are in general less sexually active than men in long-term relationships – even if they don't feel sexual enough. So breaking up is not the path to more sex. Just the opposite... until you get into a new relationship.

Break-ups are hard, no doubt about it. Some are necessary for the person who does the leaving, or for couples who mutually agree to end things. But before breaking up, I would urge people to get some counselling and make a good-faith effort to patch things up, if possible. After all, you did fall in love once, long ago.

Women tend to tell their troubles to friends. Men tend to withdraw – into silence or substance abuse. That's why men often (not always, but often) have a harder time with break-ups than women. They often don't have as much of a social support network to help them through the dark tunnel of mourning, and then to help them meet someone new.

My advice to men whose relationships end – especially for those who are broken-up-upon: work hard not to increase your alcohol consumption, or use of any other recreational, mood-altering drugs. Identify a few friends and/or family members and talk with them frequently for the first several months. Get in touch with a few old friends and talk with them. Consider professional counselling as well. When you're over the worst of it, and you start to think about dating again, do things you consider fun and try to meet people that way. Join a new club. Take up a new hobby. That sort of thing.

Monogamy

I take a Darwinian view of sex. Men have the greatest chance of genetic survival if they spread their seed far and wide. Women have the greatest chance of genetic survival if they nurture their children with the help of an able mate. I know this doesn't explain everything, but for me, it goes a long way towards explaining why most men have more problems with monogamy than most women do.

Monogamy is not 'natural' for men, and many, many men chafe under it. On the other hand, monogamy (actually serial monogamy) is our cultural norm. For better or worse, it's the way Western society is organised. And it certainly beats wondering if your spouse is coming home to you every night. I've made my personal peace with monogamy. It's not perfect, but in the context of our culture, it beats the alternative. The challenge for couples is to keep things romantic and erotic, which takes constant work and creativity. But it can be fun, too.

Celibacy

As an adult, I have never been voluntarily celibate. People are sexual. I am a sexual person. It's a part of life I enjoy, value and consider important. I've been with the same woman 30 years. We have had our sexual ups and downs as all couples do, but we have never stopped being sexual with one another.

If people decide to be celibate for a while, that's fine. Many women in recovery from sexual abuse find that a period of celibacy helps them come to terms with their abuse history and eventually overcome it. So celibacy has its uses. But personally, I've never had much use for it.

Bill O'Hanlon

Having a good relationship

That is a complex question and one that is different for different relationships. If I had to say what I have experienced and observed as a generalisation, I would say that an acceptance of the other person and their differences is a key ingredient of a good relationship. Simone Weil said some years ago something like it is fairly easy to love someone, but to love them with their desires, especially when what they desire is not what you would want them to desire, is much more difficult. I and my wife, Steffanie, have called that 'radical acceptance'.

Monogamy

I'm not certain if there is a difference in being monogamous for men and women. In therapy, I certainly hear that for women, it seems much more about being listened to, respected and heard than just about sexual variety much of the time, but again this is not universal.

Celibacy

In my model of therapy, something is only a problem if someone is complaining about it or it physically harms someone, so I wouldn't say celibacy per se is a problem. I would help someone who was making that choice come to see it as OK and not shameful or sick. If it were occurring in a couple relationship and both partners were OK with it, again I would help them withstand others'/society's critiques and judgements. If one partner were dissatisfied, then it becomes a couple's problem and I have no formulaic way to deal with that. It would require conversation and consideration for each unique situation.

Dominic Davies

Having a good relationship
Listen to your partner with an open heart.

Practise random acts of kindness.

Say what's in your heart, spend time each week sharing something of your soul.

Monogamy
I think monogamy is a patriarchal capitalist concept creating property and ownership out of people's love. It also shores up low self-esteem, but does nothing to deal with the root cause. If you really love someone, why wouldn't you want him or her to be all they can be? To grow in the direction of their choice, even if it means without you. This is love.

Celibacy
I think there's a distinction between choosing not to be sexual, either with oneself or others, and wanting to, but not being able to have sex. I see the first as celibacy and the latter as potentially problematic, and perhaps it may help to seek out someone to talk to about it.

George Taleporos

Celibacy
I have been single and very much celibate for all of my life. I think the most important thing is valuing yourself in the absence of a sexual relationship – that is something that many people struggle with, whether they have or do not have a physical disability. Sexual relationships can be very rewarding, but so can a single life. After all, you have more time for your friends, for your work and for yourself – recognising these benefits can be very helpful for a person who has been single

for a long time. Remember that being celibate does not mean that you are asexual. In my study [see Chapter 8], over 40 per cent of the participants did not have a sexual partner, but they were certainly very sexual people.

Eugene Moore

Having a good relationship & monogamy

A good relationship comes from regarding love as a verb – as something that one does, as opposed to regarding love as a state of being – as something that one is 'in'. History helps unravel the puzzle.

In a nutshell, the notion of 'being in love' was popularised by the troubadours of the medieval French royal court. Romantic love was put forth as the premier type of relationship between two people – seeing the other person as an ideal type, and being 'lost' in a state of perpetual infatuation. But this could only be maintained if real life did not enter the picture. The troubadours knew that such idealism could not survive day-to-day life, and so the notion of being in love required that the relationship be kept in the realm of fantasy.

That was all well and good, until the circumstances of history turned everything upside down. As the ideal of romantic love filtered from the royal court to the masses over the centuries, people began to accept 'being in love' as the ideal type of relationship. In the meantime, social changes in Europe led to a decline in arranged marriages based upon social and economic considerations. People began to choose their own partners – and of course, they began to choose those partners on the basis of the new ideal of 'being in love'.

This is when a temporary phenomenon (being 'in love') was attached to a real-life permanent relationship (marriage or co-habitation). Thus, we have come to believe that the ideal is to 'fall in love' with someone and that the natural outcome is to pair up with that person in a real-life relationship. The problem comes when the fantasy flies away in the face of reality, and we are no longer 'in love' with the person, with the natural outcome being to split up and 'fall in love' with someone else to start the whole thing over again.

It is not that 'falling in love' will never form the basis for a good and lasting relationship. The problem is that instead of concentrating on 'being' loving – that is, on behaving towards our partner with acts of caring and love (love as a verb) – we find ourselves concentrating on maintaining a 'state of being' (love as an adjective) whose reality we base upon having certain 'feelings'. 'We've lost that lovin' feelin', now it's gone, gone, gone' goes the song. And as the feeling goes, so does the relationship.

Love that keeps people together in happiness is not an adjective that describes a blissful state of being – it is a verb that describes actions. The really interesting thing is that when one regards love as a verb, then the power to create love is in the hands of the lover. All I have to do to create love is to decide to 'do' loving things. When love is a state of being, then I am at its mercy – it comes and it goes and is out of my control, as in the above song.

And it is not as if treating love as a verb means that the relationship is devoid of loving feelings – on the contrary. It would be very difficult for two people who are committed to acting lovingly towards each other to not experience deep and abiding feelings for each other. But the feelings follow from the actions – not from some fanciful 'condition' popularised by French poets and sought desperately by millions of people who assume that 'being in love' describes an elusive reality for which they spend their lives searching.

Take a look at good relationships around you – I'll bet that whether or not the partners understand the difference between love as a verb and as an adjective, the former is a daily reality.

Celibacy

When couples go through times when they aren't sexual it must be realised that there is little chance that the overwhelming sexual excitement that often characterises new relationships can remain over time. That has nothing to do with the love in the relationship – it is just that making love to the same 'body' over and over for years is bound to lose some of its 'edge'. I think a lot of couples simply become great friends, and the sexual side may just slowly fade away or become less intense.

Reverend Bill Huff Johnston

Having a good relationship

I like lots of mystery, humour and play in my relationships. Communication, direct honesty is important. I am in favour of the explicit, of being honest and straightforward. Follow these rules: if we love someone, we tell them; if there is someone we can't stand, keep out of their way; and if there is someone in between, keep an open mind. Remember: 'There but for the love of God, go I.' Be open to a smile across a crowded room, and keep the surprise in your relationship.

Monogamy

I think it is almost impossible to be monogamous if we love other human beings and if we give expression to our love (it doesn't have to be sexual but there is choice). There are some times when it is right to say 'yes' and there are some times when it is right to say 'no', or change our minds. What we feel and what we do are not necessarily the same thing.

I feel that men may be less sensitive, thoughtful and fearful than women and that women are more cautious and more careful. It will also be different depending on what age we are, be it in our twenties, thirties, forties, fifties or sixties. Passion remains the same, but priorities change.

Celibacy
This is not something I would choose, but I recognise that for many it is their strength. I believe that there should be choice and I do not judge people on their choice. I think that this would be a very difficult decision because it would bring up many frustrations. However, the times I go on retreat are rich times because they bring out many positive things.

Rabbi Shmuley Boteach

Having a good relationship
Complete and constant communication is essential. Every marriage or relationship needs a constant element of surprise, because if you let your marriage fall into a routine, chances are it will die, or at least become so stultifyingly boring that you wish it would die. From my experience, the way to stop being bored is for partners to keep wooing each other and never to take each other for granted.

Monogamy
Of course it is hard to be monogamous, especially for men, more than for women. But it is a good thing in a way, because since men need constant excitement due to their nature, they can bring constant excitement into the relationship. If men can just use their non-monogamous nature in order to be monogamous, then they are constantly creating fireworks for a woman. They are now exploring every sexual possibility with her and making her feel incredibly desirable because they are having to cater to their own need for variety.

Celibacy
I don't think celibacy is a natural state. It is like saying that someone doesn't want to eat. Of course, people go on fasts, and people can get used to less, but it is still not healthy. Sex is a

necessity, and not for procreative reasons. Sex is a necessity because it is the ultimate affirmation that a person in their naked passive state is still desirable and is still an object of love. And if someone wants to make love to you, that affirms you and makes you feel alive. There are two great human needs: to feel alive and to feel understood. Sex is the solution to both. Sex literally makes you feel more alive. Your blood races faster and you become hotter – literally. Heat and the pulse are the measurements of how alive we are.

Second, sex makes you feel understood because you divest yourself of all artificial layers, and your core is exposed. And when you feel that your core is exposed, that you are vulnerable, but nevertheless, you are still accepted and loved, you can't be lonely, because in your innermost depths someone has been joined on to you.

The human being is comprised of two different parts – the body and the soul. The body needs to feel alive – affirmation of the sexual, and the soul needs to feel understood, to feel connected. Hence passion and intimacy are the two great human needs, and both are provided for in a healthy sexual relationship. Celibacy undermines all that.

Winton Higgins

Having a good relationship

A very famous Thai meditation master often had newlyweds come to him for advice about how to make their marriage successful. His advice was simple: practise the basic Buddhist precepts with each other. In other words, if we constantly try to lift our game with each other, and the game is about love, generosity, care in sexual matters, honesty and mental clarity, we can't go wrong. All those thick, complicated 'how to' books either say this, in which case they're superfluous, or say something different, in which case they're wrong.

Monogamy

Buddhism doesn't see monogamy as inherently virtuous, but let's assume we choose it anyway. Anyone who is a hostage to the Advertising Agency's View of Life will find monogamy virtually impossible to practise. This is because the reality is that we're constantly surrounded by alluring bipeds, so go for it – acquire and consume them! By contrast, anyone who is a free and self-understanding agent will know that saying 'no' is often the essence of freedom. Practising monogamy doesn't depend on repression, but on awareness of who we are, where we stand and what's really going on.

Celibacy

All sorts of situations arise in our lives when a capacity for contented celibacy can enrich us, and certainly steer us clear of a lot of unnecessary suffering and destructiveness. Some people choose celibacy as part of a long- or short-term commitment to intense spiritual practice, as monastics or when on retreat. Sometimes in lay life our partner is away or unavailable. In no case does a celibate cease to be a sexual being.

The biological drive and the cultural trumpeting of sex are always there. Celibacy is an ideal opportunity to attend to these elements in our lives. Will I really need an operation if I don't get so-many orgasms a week? Is the culturally induced obsession with sex contributing to my wellbeing, or should I just let it go through to the keeper (as cricketers say)?

The human mind possesses a simple, powerful mechanism that Buddhist practice depends on. Given enough stillness and space, the mind will recognise what *really* contributes to its wellbeing and what only creates suffering. It will then quite instinctively, in the Buddha's term, 'incline towards' what contributes to wellbeing. The rest it will gently but confidently send to the dump, where it belongs – including the Advertising Agency's View of Life.

Sex

Never repress it!
Never be against it.
Rather, go deep into it
with great clarity,
with great love.
Go like an explorer.
Search all the nooks and corners
of your sexuality,
and you will
be surprised and
enriched and benefited.
Knowing your sexuality,
one day you will
stumble upon your
spirituality.
Then you will be free.
The future will have
a totally different
vision of sex.
It will be
more fun, more joy,
more friendship,
more a play than
a serious affair
as it has been in the past.
Sex is just
the beginning,
not the end.
But if you miss the beginning,
you will miss
the end also.

(*Tantra, Spirituality & Sex*, Osho)

Further Information

Contacts

Chapter 1

Joseph Kramer: e-mail: kramer@erospirit.org
Web sites: www.erospirit.org and www.eroticmassage.com
PO Box 3893, Oakland, CA 94609, USA

Mantak Chia: Web site: www.healing-tao.com/master

Stan Dale: Web site: www.hai.org

Chapter 2

Willem de Ridder: e-mail: wdridder@xs4all.nl
Web site: www.willemderidder.com

Keith Hennessy: Web site: www.848.com

Panos Couros: Web site: homepages.ihug.com.au~panos

Chapter 3

Shai Shahar: Web sites: come.to/coracoracora and members.ams.chello.nl/c.e.emens/Shai.html

Dan Savage: Web site: www.thestranger.com

Chapter 4

Richard Pacheco: e-mail: bardook@earthlink.net

Robbie Swan: Web site: www.eros.org.au

Chapter 5

Layne Winklebleck: Web site: www.spectator.net

Robert McGinley: e-mail: rm@nasca.com

Chapter 6

David Steinberg: Web site: www.sexuality.org/davids.html

Kenneth Ray Stubbs: Web site: www.sexandspirit.com
Tel: (001) 520 743 8100 ext. 102
5631 West Placita, Del Risco Dep M, Tucson, Arizona 85745, USA

Kerry Riley: 'Tantric Goddess' sessions in Australia or the US, contact: Spectra 2000 Pty Ltd, PO Box 97, Avalon Beach, NSW 2107, Australia. Tel: (0061) 2 9974 4724; e-mail: loveworks@ozemail.com.au

Chapter 7

Dr Jules Black: 2 Rae Street, Randwick, NSW 2031, Australia. Office tel: (0061) 2 9398 1888; fax: (0061) 2 9326 5717

David Brown: Web site: www.icasa.co.uk

Michael Castleman: Web sites: www.Xandria.com; wwwOnHealth.com; SelfCare.com; Depression.com; Alzheimers.com

Bill O'Hanlon: Possibilities, 551 W. Cordova Rd, #715, Santa Fe, New Mexico 87501, USA. Tel: (001) 505 983 2843; fax (001) 505 983 2761; Web site: www.brieftherapy.com

Chapter 8

Dominic Davies: e-mail: serene@dircon.co.uk and ACCSEX-subscribe@yahoogroups.com

George Taleporos: e-mail: gtdeakin@bigpond.net.au

Eugene Moore: Web site: www.fullspectrum.co.nz

Chapter 9

Reverend Bill Huff Johnston: Web site: www.eros.org.au

Rabbi Shmuley Boteach: e-mail: shmuley@healtheworld.com

Winton Higgins: e-mail: brusan@ihug.com.au

Bibliography

Gibran, K (1996) *The Prophet*, Wordsworth Editions, London

His Holiness the Dalai Lama (1995) *The World of Tibetan Buddhism*, translated, edited and annotated by Dr Thupten Jinpa, Wisdom Publications

Krishnamurti, K (1997) *The First and Last Freedom*, HarperSanFrancisco, San Francisco, CA

Osho (formally known as Bhagwan Shree Rajneesh) (1983) *Tantra, Spirituality & Sex*, Rajneesh Foundation International, Oregon, US

About the Author

Jo-Anne Baker was the first person to introduce futon mattresses to Australia in the early 1980s. After revolutionising the bedding industry she is now well known as one of Australia's leading sex entrepreneurs, therapists and educators. Her business, The Pleasure Spot, was established in 1993 and was one of the first businesses in Australia to focus on women's and couples' sexuality, specialising in courses and products.

Jo-Anne now concentrates on her private sessions. She draws on her training in sociology, psychology, bio-energetics, hypnotherapy, meditation, tantra and erotic spirituality.

She is the author of *Self Sexual Healing: Finding Pleasure Within* and the editor of *Sex Tips From Women Who Ride the Sexual Frontier*, both published by Fusion Press.

Jo-Anne can be contacted via e-mail at: pleaspot@ozemail.com.au.

Her Web site is: www.pleasurespot.com.au.